PAIN, PLEASURE, AND AMERICAN CHILDBIRTH

Contributions in Medical History

PAIN, PLEASURE, AND AMERICAN CHILDBIRTH

From the Twilight Sleep to the Read Method, 1914–1960

Margarete Sandelowski

CONTRIBUTIONS IN MEDICAL HISTORY, NUMBER 13

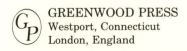

GREENWOOD PRESS
Westport, Connecticut
London, England

Library of Congress Cataloging in Publication Data

Sandelowski, Margarete.
  Pain, pleasure, and American childbirth.

  (Contributions in medical history, ISSN 0147-1058 ;
no. 13)
  Bibliography: p.
  Includes index.
  1. Childbirth—United States—History—20th century.
2. Natural childbirth—United States—History—20th
century.   3. Pain.   4. Childbirth—Psychological
aspects.   I. Title.   II. Series.
RG652.S243   1984   618.4'5   83-18510
ISBN 0-313-24076-0 (lib. bdg.)

Library of Congress Catalog Card Number: 83-18510
ISBN: 0-313-24076-0
ISSN: 0147-1058

First published in 1984

Greenwood Press
A division of Congressional Information Service, Inc.
88 Post Road West, Westport, Connecticut 06881

Printed in the United States of America

10 9 8 7 6 5 4 3 2 1

For Leslie and Nadia

CONTENTS ———————————

ACKNOWLEDGMENTS _____

This study was funded, in part, by a National Research Service Nurse Fellowship Award from the Department of Health and Human Services, Public Health Service, Health Resources Administration, Bureau of Health Professions and by a Graduate Alumni Award from Case Western Reserve University. I thank the staffs of the following libraries and especially Glen Jenkins of the Historical Division of the Cleveland Health Sciences Library and Lenore Maxa; Susan Alon and Ferencz Gyorgyey of the Yale Medical History Library; and Esther Hanchett of the Library of the Maternity Center Association of New York. I also thank Margaret Thoms for sharing her father's letters, Dr. Morrell Heald for his cheerful encouragement, Dr. Rosemary Ellis for maintaining standards of excellence just out of my reach, Dr. Darwin Stapleton for his perceptive and gentle criticism, Betty Suber for her unfailing kindness, and Dr. Linda Kirby because. . . .

INTRODUCTION ————————

In 1927, when Edith Wharton published her novel, *Twilight Sleep*, many women "drifted into motherhood . . . lightly and unperceivingly."[1] The "beauty" of birth-giving lay in feeling and remembering nothing at all about it. By 1949, the "pleasure" of childbirth lay in savoring every one of its sensations, even its pain.[2] What happened to alter Americans' views of beauty and pleasure in childbirth and whether any substantive change really occurred at all are the subjects of this book.

Pain, Pleasure, and American Childbirth describes the evolution of American childbirth, namely, the shift in emphasis from the conquest of pain to the quest for pleasure. It traces Americans' views and practice of childbirth from the Twilight Sleep through the early Natural Childbirth movements within the framework of pain and pleasure. In addition, it analyzes the consequences this relatively recent shift had for the trajectory of labor, for the relationships among childbearing women, nurses, and physicians, and for the conceptualization of childbirth and women.

The subject of pain is an integral part of any analysis of American childbirth practices. Arguably the most important event in the history of American childbirth occurred when physicians, eager to obtain the right to attend women in childbirth, promised them relief from pain; and women, eager to be relieved of pain, turned to physicians to fulfill that promise.

Until the 1940s, American childbirth practices were largely informed by the desire to alleviate pain. As the phenomenon Americans most closely associated with childbirth, pain crystallized all of the potential hazards of childbirth and served as a focus for professionals' and women's fear of it. Linked in their minds with suffering, injury, and death, pain apparently defined childbirth.

Prior to 1914, the major "pain task"[3] assumed primarily by childbearing women was to *endure* pain. A general feeling prevailed that labor pain was both inevitable and necessary and therefore ought not to be relieved. In addition, few reliable and safe remedies for pain relief in labor existed, and a combination of factors, including physician skill and patient social class, served to limit the use of available pharmacologic measures for pain relief.

After 1915, when the Twilight Sleep debate finally demonstrated that pain was dangerous in labor and that it could be successfully alleviated, *relief* emerged as the major pain task. Between 1915 and 1948, physicians and nurses assumed the major responsibility for dealing with labor pain as women increasingly transferred their own responsibility for pain relief to professionals and as physicians, in particular, recognized the professional advantages of assuming that obligation. Moreover, physicians relied almost exclusively on drugs that induced amnesia or the complete obliteration of sensation in labor and on drugs and instruments that paradoxically inflicted pain, both as means to abate the natural pain of labor. The task of relief clearly included the task of *inflicting* pain.

By 1948, with the advent of the Natural Childbirth "craze," a new impetus for the conduct of American childbirth appeared along with the desire to alleviate pain, and that was the desire to enhance pleasure. Pleasure—or satisfaction or happiness—was viewed as something more than and different from what a woman experienced from mere pain relief. That is, pleasure was not simply the opposite of pain. Natural Childbirth promised a happy experience of birth-giving by emphasizing the tasks of *preventing* and *minimizing* pain. Pain could be prevented by instilling fearlessness in women through education and intensive training, and it could be minimized .

by severing the mental association between pain and what women felt in childbirth. Natural Childbirth also promised that even if a woman felt her labor as pain, she could still derive pleasure from it. Words such as ecstasy and exhilaration began to accompany and even replace pain as descriptions of childbirth as women now experienced it. Moreover, women reassumed much, if not most, of the burden for dealing with labor pain. The table on pp. xiv–xv summarizes the pain tasks, agents, means, and underlying views of pain that evolved over time.[4]

Pain, Pleasure, and Childbirth

Women and men have always found it hard to comprehend and to convey to each other what they feel experiencing childbirth and what they see witnessing it. This problem of understanding and communication is, in large part, due to the difficulty in defining the phenomenon most commonly associated with childbirth, namely, pain. For Margaret Mead, pain is a "form of human experience so sharp, so unmistakable, so immediate, that members of any culture can recognize, empathize, or identify with another human being in pain."[5] In contrast, others have observed how easy it is for human beings to mistake fear, exhaustion, violent effort, pleasure, and even ecstasy—phenomena associated with pain—for pain itself. They emphasize the private and incommunicable aspects of the pain experience. None of us can feel another person's pain. We can only feel what another person must be feeling.[6]

In short, underlying the problem of defining pain is the use of a single word to refer to a personal and unshared experience of hurting, suffering, or anguish (what is pain to you is not pain to me, or your pain can never be like mine); a patterned and shared cultural response protecting a group of individuals from harm (when in pain, cry, isolate yourself, see a doctor, for example); as well as any warning stimulus signaling current or impending injury (from the urge to void to the sensations of a heart attack).[7]

These definitions reveal that pain is both subjective and objective, both particular and universal, and both helpful and

Table: 1 The View of Pain, Its Tasks, Alleviating Agents and Means, 1847–1960

	1847–1914	1914–1948	1948–1960
major pain task	to endure	· to relieve · to inflict	· to prevent · to minimize
agent primarily responsible for major pain task	childbearing woman	professional caregiver	cooperative effort between childbearing woman and caregiver
secondary pain task	enable endurance	transfer pain responsibility	
secondary agent	professional and family caregivers		
means to achieve pain tasks	· personal resources of woman · "emotional support" and physical comfort · intermittent and brief pharmacologic analgesia and anesthesia	pharmacologically induced amnesia, semi- to complete unconsciousness, and regional obliteration of labor sensations	· mental reindoctrination · physical reconditioning · breathing and relaxation techniques · "emotional support" and physical comfort · intermittent and brief pharmacologic analgesia and

view of childbirth pain	• expected • functional • inevitable	• expected • dysfunctional • treatable • emphasized physiologic origins of pain and pain as a technical problem	anesthesia and local obliteration of labor sensation • as "credit" for future pleasure • not necessarily expected at all • functional • preventable • emphasized psychogenic origins of pain and pain as an emotional problem

harmful. Moreover, pain is a concept that can be conveyed in a number of different languages. In the language of neuro-physiology, pain is a quantifiable sensation. In the language of psychology, pain is a qualitative affective state. In the everyday languages of people, pain is, among other things, an evil, a punishment, a burden, and a challenge.

Observers of Western people—Americans, in particular—have noted their virtual obsession with avoiding or relieving pain and demonstrating their highly negative view of it.[8] Social critic Ivan Illich argued that "medical civilization" made pain intolerable by detaching it from a meaningful context and by depicting it as "curable." Believing that persons deprived of the responsibility for dealing with their own pain are also deprived of an "uniquely human performance called suffering," Illich condemned the Western "killing of pain" with drugs that turned people who used to be able to cope with the harsh realities of life into "anesthesia consumers" desperate to escape them.[9]

In a similar but less urgent vein, anthropologist Mark Zborowski remarked that Americans focus their efforts relative to pain on avoiding it.[10] American physician Walter Modell cited pain as the most common of complaints and the one that, in American culture, "invokes the promptest and most pressing demand for relief." Maintaining that pain had no "virtue" to Americans, except in cases where an individual willingly endured pain not to give information to an enemy or to be "beautiful," Modell indicated that "relief" is an important part of the American "culture of comfort" and the physician's main reason for being.[11]

Women's experiences in childbirth present distinctive problems in understanding and communication because of the pain-pleasure dilemma that giving birth evokes. For centuries, philosophers, theologians, physicians, and scientists have debated whether pain and pleasure are two distinct and opposing entities or different manifestations of the same sensation, experience, or passion. It has also been debated whether a single experience can provide both pain and pleasure and whether normal people can derive pleasure from pain.[12]

Women's childbearing experiences have appeared in the

contexts of the religious martyr for whom the agony of self-inflicted or sought-after wounds and dying are ecstasy; of the man for whom the confrontation with war is painful but satisfying; of the athlete who chooses to obtain a "high" from driving mind and body to the limits of endurance; and even of the masochist who can only derive pleasure from pain.[13] While these pain-pleasure experiences do not adequately account for the choices and constraints involved in childbirth and motherhood, they do underscore the extremely divergent views of childbirth that exist.

Until fairly recently, most published accounts of childbirth depicted it as a painful and potentially hazardous experience. In contrast, the very few real and fictional accounts of childbirth written by women themselves indicate that they do not find it incongruous to speak of childbirth in the dual contexts of life and death, exaltation and terror, reward and punishment, and pleasure and pain. For women, childbirth can include "pain" and "ecstasy." The moment of birth can be "terrific" and "like death." The sensations of labor can be "extraordinary" but painful when "fought and resisted."[14] From their descriptions, birth is at once a natural, ordinary, life-giving, and growth-promoting experience *and* a supernatural event, extraordinary, miraculous, and like dying. It is at once exciting, like a climax, *and* an agony, a mutilation, and a violation. For women, pain gives form to the dangers of childbirth and the constraints of motherhood, while pleasure gives form to the sensuality and promise of maternity. Describing childbirth in terms of pain and pleasure is capturing the ways women make sense of the experience.[15]

Notes

1. Edith Wharton, *Twilight Sleep* (New York: D. Appleton, 1927),   •
p. 14.

2. B. M. McKinney, "The Pleasure of Childbirth," *Ladies Home Journal*, April 1949, pp. 116, 118–20.

3. Shizuko Y. Fagerhaugh and Anselm Strauss, *Politics of Pain Management: Staff-Patient Interaction* (Menlo Park, Calif.: Addison-Wesley, 1977), p. 244.

4. This overview is not intended as a definitive periodization of the history of pain in American childbirth but rather as a useful one for capturing changes. These are detailed in the text.

5. Margaret Mead, foreword to *People in Pain*, by Mark Zborowski (San Francisco: Jossey-Bass, 1969), p. ix.

6. David Bakan, *Disease, Pain, and Suffering: Toward A Psychology of Suffering* (Chicago: University of Chicago Press, 1968); George W. Crile, *The Origins and Nature of the Emotions: Miscellaneous Papers* (Philadelphia: W. B. Saunders, 1915), see photos on pp. 162 and 165; and Richard A. Sternbach, *Pain: A Psychophysiological Analysis* (New York: Academic Press, 1968), p. 1.

7. Crile, *Origins and Nature of the Emotions*, pp. 77–90; Richard Serjeant, *The Spectrum of Pain* (London: Rupert Hart-Davis, 1969); and Sternbach, *Pain*, p. 12.

8. See the discussion of the American "hospital" culture in Donald Meyer, *The Positive Thinkers: A Study of the American Quest for Health, Wealth, and Personal Power from Mary Baker Eddy to Norman Vincent Peale* (New York: Doubleday, 1965), p. 17.

9. Ivan Illich, *Medical Nemesis: The Expropriation of Health* (New York: Random House, 1976), pp. 133–54.

10. Zborowski, *People in Pain*, p. 43.

11. Walter Modell, *Relief of Symptoms*, 2nd ed. (St. Louis: C. V. Mosby, 1961), pp. 13–15, 38, 75–77.

12. J. L. Cowan, *Pleasure and Pain: A Study in Philosophical Psychology* (New York: St. Martin's Press, 1968); H. Mersky and F. G. Spear, *Pain: Psychological and Psychiatric Aspects* (London: Baillere, Tindall and Cassell, 1967), pp. 3–13; Daniel De Moulin, "A Historical-Phenomenological Study of Bodily Pain in Western Man," *Bulletin of the History of Medicine* 48 (Winter 1974):540–70; P. Procacci, "History of the Pain Concept," in *Pain and Society*, ed. H. W. Kosterlitz and L. Y. Terenius (Weinheim: Verlag Chemie GmbH., 1980), pp. 3–12; and Thomas S. Szasz, *Pain and Pleasure: A Study of Bodily Feelings* (New York: Basic Books, 1957).

13. M. Beatrice Blankenship, "The Enduring Miracle," *Atlantic Monthly*, October 1933, pp. 409–15; Helene Deutsch, *The Psychology of Women Volume II. Motherhood* (1945; reprint ed., New York: Bantam, 1973), pp. 253–71; Marjorie Karmel, *Thank You, Dr. Lamaze: A Mother's Experiences in Painless Childbirth* (Philadelphia: J. B. Lippincott, 1959); and Charlotte Teller, "The Neglected Psychology of the Twilight Sleep," *Good Housekeeping*, July 1915, p. 18.

14. Enid Bagnold, *The Door of Life* (New York: William Morrow,

1938), pp. 106–7, 153–54, and McKinney, "Pleasure of Childbirth," p. 116.

15. Kathleen L. Norr et al., "Explaining Pain and Enjoyment in Childbirth," *Journal of Health and Social Behavior* 18 (September 1977):260–62. For other woman-derived descriptions of childbirth, see Gwendolyn Brooks, *Maud Martha* (New York: Harper and Brothers, 1951), pp. 89–99; Rosellen Brown, *The Autobiography of My Mother* (New York: Ballantine, 1976), p. 26; Margaret Jarman Hagood, *Mothers of the South: Portraiture of the White Tenant Farm Woman* (1939; reprint ed., New York: W. W. Norton, 1977), pp. 108–27; and Ann Oakley, *Women Confined: Towards a Sociology of Childbirth* (New York: Schocken Books, 1980). The last two texts contain direct quotations from women concerning childbirth.

PAIN,
PLEASURE,
AND AMERICAN
CHILDBIRTH

1 _____

THE CONQUEST OF PAIN: RIDING THE TWILIGHT SLEEPING CAR _____

If the many requests for information about and the demand for painless childbirth that followed the June 1914 *McClure's* article on the subject are any indication, many women viewed childbirth as unnecessarily painful.[1] In the article, Marguerite Tracy and Constance Leupp described the Twilight Sleep method of providing pain relief in labor that had been introduced and developed in Germany. Designed for "wiping the whole incident of birth-giving out of a woman's life," the Twilight Sleep was a state of semiconsciousness induced by morphine and scopolamine.[2]

The Twilight Sleep attracted many women as staunch advocates. One of them, Hanna Rion Ver Beck, summarized an essentially middle-and upper-class view of childbirth when she stated that it was a woman's "greatest hour of trial" and that the pain of childbirth, like all pain, was "destructive, disintegrating, inharmonious, undermining, unnatural, [and] unnecessary."[3] In her book about the Twilight Sleep, Ver Beck noted that childbirth was the only physiologic event in life accompanied by "great suffering."[4] Indicating that upper-class women were particularly sensitive to the nervous shock that resulted from intense suffering, she stated that pain and the fear of pain in childbirth had made many of these woman virtual neurasthenic invalids. Moreover, pain and the fear associated with it caused suffering in the husbands who witnessed their agony as well as morbid effects in their unborn children. Accordingly, pain and the fear of it had to be eliminated for the health and welfare of women, men, and children. Ver Beck implied that if that meant obliterating the experience of childbirth itself from the consciousness of women by a medicial regimen such as the Twilight Sleep, the loss to women would be negligible and the benefit to women and society enormous.

Other women advocates of the Twilight Sleep agreed with Ver Beck that pain in childbirth was unnatural and, therefore, physically and psychologically dangerous to women and infants. Mary Sumner Boyd, herself a Twilight Sleep mother, compared the risks of childbirth with those men faced in war.[5] Indicating that men only confronted the pain, anguish, and death associated with war perhaps once in a generation, while women faced these in childbirth all the time, Boyd hailed the Twilight Sleep as the promise of freedom from the nine-month ordeal of fear in pregnancy and from the many hours of pain in childbirth.

Indeed, Boyd's views indicate the extent to which the Twilight Sleep was perceived as liberating women from the restraints and mortal hazards imposed on them by their bodies. In an era when American women, such as Tracy, Leupp, and Boyd, were actively and publicly seeking the rights and privileges long denied to their sex, it was not surprising that they would also "rebel against enduring the usual tortures and miseries of childbirth," which, in their opinion, weakened women for the struggle to obtain those rights.[6]

Women advocates of the Twilight Sleep suggested that an important measure of a woman's freedom was her ability to escape the handicap of childbearing. Tracy and Boyd clarified the strong connection between women's quest for painless childbirth and their quest for equality with men by asserting that the fear of pain in childbirth alone had probably been a "potent factor in retarding [women's] development to a position of equality with men."[7] Reiterating the view that men, except in war and in some dangerous trades, did not have to face the constant threat to life and health that women were forced to confront in maternity, Tracy and Boyd indicated that women bore the greater burden of the world's pain. The Twilight Sleep was, accordingly, a vital means to equalize women's and men's share of suffering since it allowed women to subtract the ordeal of labor and delivery—the period of maternity most dreaded by women.

Twilight Sleep advocates revealed the desperation and even anger with which women of their class seemed to approach the prospect of giving birth. For these women, childbirth sapped a woman's will, caused her needless physical and mental trauma, interfered with her efforts to take her rightful place in the world alongside men, and even killed her.

Women such as Tracy, Leupp, Boyd, and Ver Beck believed that men did not fully appreciate the difficulties inherent in maternity and that physicians, in particular, were ignorant of or had deliberately withheld the means by which the problem of pain in labor could be solved. While these writers still viewed maternity as a woman's greatest asset in achieving power and influence in society, they viewed childbirth, which they equated with pain, mutilation, and death, as her greatest liability. The very zeal with which Twilight Sleep advocates promoted the method underscored how important they believed maternity was, not only to women but also to the preservation of the family and society. For these women, the fear of childbirth marred the experience of pregnancy, and the trauma induced by childbirth marred the experience of motherhood. Accordingly, if a woman had to submit her body to childbirth in order to become a mother, with the Twilight Sleep, she did not have to submit her mind.

In the early decades of the twentieth century, women still had good reason to associate childbirth with pain and death. First, not all women who may have wanted available pharmacologic pain-relieving methods received them, and, second, it was commonplace for women and infants to be injured in childbirth or die of maternity-related causes.

Prior to 1847, most women were resigned to pain in labor because there were so few reliable remedies to alleviate it. If soporific agents such as opiates and alcohol were used at all, they tended to stop labor or drug the infant when given ineffective analgesic doses. Moreover, such pain-relieving remedies as blood-letting and purgation were themselves causes of

considerable anguish. By the middle of the nineteenth century, there had yet to be discovered a method of pain relief
that could alleviate the laboring woman's suffering but not in-
terfere with the powers of labor or harm the woman or her
child. While attempts were made to relieve it, including drugs,
potions, and forms of "mesmerism," none of them was dependable in terms of both safety and effectiveness in the vast majority of labor cases.[8]

Accordingly, the introduction of chemical anesthesia into
obstetric practice in 1847 promised a simple and certain method
of pain relief in labor, which prominent physicians advocated
and women appeared to want.[9] Yet the general Anglo-American
medical community's response to the use of agents such as ether
and chloroform demonstrated an even greater reluctance on
the part of physicians to use them in obstetrics than in surgery.[10]

This reluctance was in great part due to what was perceived as the naturalness of childbirth pain as opposed to the
artificiality of surgical pain. More precisely, surgical pain was
inflicted by a human agent and was, therefore, properly subject to human attempts at relief. In contrast, childbirth pain
was viewed as both an integral and necessary part of a normal, natural phenomenon and as a divinely ordained punishment that all women had to endure to atone for Eve's
transgressions in the garden. Childbirth pain was, therefore,
not properly subject to human intervention.[11]

The physicians (and clergymen) who joined the mid-
nineteenth-century debate about chemical anesthesia were
concerned about the medical, psychological, moral, and spiritual consequences of interfering with natural law or divine will.
They argued against anesthesia saying that it was not safe for
the mother or child and that childbirth pain was necessary to
the physiological course of labor, to act as a cueing device for
physicians in the proper management of labor, to the development of normal female emotions, and to the establishment
of a healthy mother-infant bond. Accordingly, many physicians felt unjustified in using chemical agents except in unusual or complicated cases of labor that required operative intervention (or man-made pain). Even so-called natural healers

who believed that labor pain was an unnatural result of defi-
cits in the female constitution advocated such remedies as diet
and exercise over the artificial remedy of drugs as the proper
means of alleviating childbirth pain.[12]

Physicians who were early advocates of chemical anesthesia
soon overcame their colleagues' major objections, and Queen
Victoria's use of chloroform in 1853 during the birth of her
eighth child helped to create a public demand for anesthesia
"à la reine."[13] Yet such factors as ease and cost of administration of chemical anesthetics, access to information about them,
and even the social class of the laboring woman herself inter-
acted to limit the numbers of women actually receiving anesthesia in childbirth.

Many physicians, for example, were reluctant to use chemical anesthesia because it required additional skill, equipment, and hands. Those physicians who did not regularly read
medical journals were unaware of the latest advances in pain
relief. Moreover, because of the prevailing belief that lower-
class women did not feel their labors so intensely as their
upper-class counterparts, only the upper class was viewed as
really in need of pain relief.[14] Finally, most women, through
the 1930s, delivered their babies at home with either nonphysician attendants, who were unlikely to use drugs in labor,[15]
or with physicians, for whom drug use was not so easy in the
home as it would become in the hospital.[16]

Pain and death have always been closely associated in the
human mind, but that association was strengthened in the
matter of childbirth when early reports on maternal and infant mortality revealed that tens of thousands of women and
infants were still dying each year in the United States as a
result of maternity. The analogy between childbirth and the
battlefield was as well-founded on statistical fact as it was on
sentiment.

Grace Meigs, in her 1917 survey of maternal mortality, the
first such study done for the Children's Bureau, cited maternity as the second leading cause of death, after tuberculosis,
in women between fifteen and forty-four years old and noted
that the United States was a particularly dangerous country
in which to have a baby. According to Meigs, only two of fif-

teen countries to which the United States was compared had higher rates of death connected with maternity. Furthermore, she indicated that while great progress had been made in reducing the incidence of death from such diseases as typhoid, diphtheria, and tuberculosis, no comparable progress had been made since the turn of the century in reducing maternal mortality. She attributed this lack of progress, in part, to the "fatalism" that infused most people's thinking about childbearing. Injury and death in childbirth were viewed as being as natural and, therefore, as inevitable as childbirth itself.[17]

Both women and physicians believed that women had become less capable over time of withstanding the ordeal of childbirth. The view of childbirth that evolved from the colonial period through the early decades of the twentieth century was that, in normal circumstances, childbirth was a painless and uncomplicated event but that there were fewer and fewer cases of childbirth that could be considered normal. In the midnineteenth century, women, especially those who were intellectually and socioeconomically favored, were often pictured as inherently weak, sickly, and overly sensitive to the effects of their unique physiological functions. Childbirth, in particular, was perceived as a tremendous shock to the female nervous system with limited energy reserves.[18]

Although women who were nonwhite, lacking in education and intelligence, or poor were viewed as requiring little or no attention at confinement, civilized women, or women in the middle and upper classes, were viewed as laboring under the "penalty of civilization and artificial refinement."[19] These refined and exquisitely sensitive women had evolved into "hothouse product[s] . . . physically less fit to perpetuate the race."[20] Modern social customs and fashion, which did not influence less refined women, had imposed upon the civilized woman an artificial way of life that interfered with her constitutional vigor. Too much mental activity diverted energy from the reproductive organs, and overly tight corsets deformed the body. In short, the modern woman who was favored by civilization, intellectually and socially, was also perceived as having been unfitted by civilization to withstand the onslaught of her physical nature. Consequently, childbirth had become an unnatural condition in the modern woman.

Both professional and lay advocates of the Twilight Sleep argued that the method allowed childbirth to be natural again. They indicated that the Twilight Sleep resulted in an easier birth because it permitted the physiological functions of the woman's reproductive system to work unimpeded by her mind. Significantly, Twilight Sleep advocates clearly separated the pain of childbirth, or the somatic sensation of labor, from the fear of childbirth, or the negative psychological context in which labor was experienced.

For example, Charlotte Teller, a Twilight Sleep mother, claimed that the method removed the "excess of thought" that weakened the refined woman in her struggle with the natural process of birth. According to Teller, the modern woman was not lacking in physical strength but rather was unduly burdened by the unconscious fear of childbirth. Drawing on the work of Freud, Teller theorized that the refined woman, not the "crude" one, needed to be unconscious during childbirth to mobilize her physical energies against the suffering and death that awaited her. The Twilight Sleep removed a woman's psychic inhibitions against childbirth so that her body could fight nature.[21]

Medical advocates of the Twilight Sleep also separated *soma* from *psyche* in the matter of childbirth pain. Bertha Van Hoosen, one of the foremost medical champions of the Twilight Sleep, believed that the method solved the problem of bearing and rearing children for the "highly organized mothers of modern civilization." By "uncoupl[ing] the brain from the spinal cord" and thus leaving the "woman a good animal to bear her offspring as easily as any other animal," the Twilight Sleep shortened labor, caused fewer lacerations and less bleeding, and resulted in a shorter period of convalescence.[22] Indeed, Van Hoosen stated, after witnessing a woman who had required forceps for a previous birth give birth to a ten-and-a-half pound infant without the aid of instruments but under the influence of the Twilight Sleep, "you begin to feel that much of the muscular effort exerted by the non-anesthetized patient was not only unnecessary, but positively wasted energy."[23]

Another early medical advocate of the Twilight Sleep, Woodbridge Hall Birchmore, noted the absence of any "inhibitory (active) resistance" on the laboring woman's part when under the influence of the method. Excited by his observations of the method, Birchmore declared that "it was as if I had seen the natural action of a woman for the first time." The Twilight Sleep restored the "truly natural conditions" of birth by allowing a woman's "natural reflexes" to predominate. It prevented her from doing " 'mischief' " to herself because of her " 'excited and voluntary or semi-voluntary actions.' " Most importantly, by sedating the "cerebrospinal axis" but not the "ganglia connected with the reflexes of common life," the Twilight Sleep effectively "stripped motherhood of its horrors."[24]

Yet, despite its apparent advantages, the Twilight Sleep was rejected by American physicians when it was first used in obstetric practice in the United States after 1906. First introduced for use in obstetrics in 1902 by a German physician, Von Steinbuchel of Graz, and subsequently refined by two other Germans, C. J. Gauss and Bernhard Kronig, the Twilight Sleep was quickly abandoned by most American physicians because of the difficulties and dangers that seemed to be inherent in the method.

The Twilight Sleep treatment, as *ideally* practiced at the Frauenklinik in Freiburg, Germany (the Freiburg technique), was begun only after labor contractions were well established in order to avoid stopping the labor before it had really begun.[25] The treatment included a first injection of 1/150 grain of scopolamine (an amnesic) with 1/2 grain of narcophin or morphine (narcotic analgesics). After forty-five minutes, a second injection of 1/150 grain of scopolamine was administered, and subsequent doses of scopolamine *only* varied according to the results of the "memory test" given to the patient.

In fact, the success of the treatment depended on the use and accurate interpretation of this test. Thirty minutes after her second dose of scopolamine, the laboring woman was asked if she had received any injections, how many and where she had received them, or she was asked if she remembered seeing an object shown to her at the time of the injection. If her memory was intact at this time, no further doses of scopolamine were given. She was, instead, tested two more times at intervals of thirty minutes. If her memory was still intact after this time, she was given an even smaller dose of scopolamine than she had received before. Again, further injections varied with the results of the memory test, which was repeated throughout the labor.

In the ideal case, the patient remained drowsy, slept between contractions, and manifested some degree of suffering during contractions. Most importantly, the patient received only as much medication as was required to keep her in an amnesic or semiconscious state in order to avoid such serious complications as infant respiratory depression at birth and uterine inertia, which prolonged labor or caused postpartum hemorrhage. Moreover, to achieve success with the Twilight Sleep, the patient had to be placed in an environment that allowed minimal visual or auditory stimulation to avoid overly exciting her during the labor and the intrusion of "memory islands," during which women recalled the pain and the events of their labors several hours after delivery. Accordingly, patients' eyes were frequently covered and their ears often blocked. They were isolated in a darkened room with professional attendants who wore costumes that made little noise as they carefully moved around the room. Even at birth, the infant was often hurried out of the delivery room, or the baby's cries were muffled by the more soothing sound of running water to ensure the relative sensory isolation of the mother.

In short, the successful Twilight Sleep treatment permitted no part of childbirth, especially pain, to mar a woman's experience of maternity. The successful Twilight Sleep mother was the woman who was completely unaware of the fact that she had borne a child until it was presented to her several hours after delivery. Since the pain of childbirth was viewed as the single most important cause of complications during and after childbirth, and since the German physicians recognized that the complete elimination of the sensation of pain could not be achieved without seriously compromising the woman, her infant, and the natural mechanism of birth, the sole objective of the Freiburg technique was that women "perceive" pain without "apperceiv[ing]" it.[26] The Twilight Sleep was not intended to eliminate the sensation of pain, which was viewed as functional, but rather to alter the laboring woman's memory of the pain, which was viewed as dysfunctional. More precisely, the

Twilight Sleep was based on the principle that it was not the pain itself that damaged women but rather women's *knowledge* of pain in childbirth.

Although American physicians after 1906 experimented with the Twilight Sleep, many of them did not adhere to the strict Freiburg technique and, consequently, wrongly attributed maternal and infant accidents in childbirth to the method. For example, some physicians began the treatment too soon; some administered repeated injections of morphine along with scopolamine; some prescribed doses of the drugs to the point of complete analgesia; and some offered the treatment in environments not conducive to its success. Few labor settings in the United States could compare with the Freiburg clinic, and busy general practitioners were reluctant to carry out every detail of the technique since that required their presence over the entire labor period instead of during the delivery phase only.[27] Moreover, there were some problems in obtaining the proper pharmaceutical preparations of morphine and scopolamine.[28]

Consequently, by 1914, most American physicians had been frightened away from the method because of its association with delayed labor, postpartum hemorrhage, and overly narcotized babies, and because it demanded a greater degree of skill and more attention than other pain-relieving methods they may have been using. Few American women were being offered the Twilight Sleep or even knew of its existence prior to the appearance of the June 1914 *McClure's* article. Yet the Twilight Sleep "furor" of 1914–1915 was created primarily by women, some of whom had experienced the Twilight Sleep themselves at the Frauenklinik and then wrote about it for magazines, gave interviews to journalists, or simply told their friends about it.

Apparently, the first American woman to have a Twilight Sleep birth was Mrs. C. Temple Emmet of New York, a granddaughter of the Astors, who happened to be in Freiburg in 1909. Pleased with the method, she returned to Germany for two more births, told her friends about the method, and eventually started the National Twilight Sleep Association in New York in 1915 to disseminate information about and agitate for the new method for the "emancipation of women from the bondage of pain."[29] Mrs. Cecil Shaw, the secretary of this organization, was also a Freiburg mother and sister of Marguerite Tracy, one of the authors of the pivotal *McClure's* article. Between 1909 and the outbreak of the First World War, a number of American women visited Freiburg to gather information about the method and to have their babies by it. Mary Boyd, for example, went to Freiburg as a journalist and as an expectant mother. She also became a member of the Twilight Sleep Association.

As suggested previously, women advocates of the Twilight Sleep were desperate to receive pain relief in labor, and they were angry with their physicians for not providing it to them. Charlotte Teller revealed the desperation by returning to Freiburg in the midst of war.[30] Boyd and Tracy revealed the anger by accusing physicians of having "killed" the Twilight Sleep just as they had killed other medical advances, such as Semmelweiss' discovery of the cause of puerperal fever.[31]

Indeed, the Twilight Sleep debate of 1914–1915 was not simply an argument about the advantages and disadvantages of a pain-relieving regimen but rather a lay revolt against what was perceived as the medical expropriation of knowledge belonging to the people. Tracy and Boyd indicated that Simpson's contribution of anesthesia to obstetric practice in the nineteenth century had been allowed to "die" because it had been "entrusted" to the medical profession. These women saw themselves as "obliged to place before the lay public of the world a gift of science which has by rights been its possession for two generations."[32] According to them, the Twilight Sleep debate represented a milestone in the history of medicine because it was the "first time . . . that the whole body of patients have risen to dictate to the doctors."[33] The Twilight Sleep furor was a democratic revolt.

By the time women such as Ver Beck and Boyd had finished their research, they knew more about the Twilight Sleep than the average medical practitioner in the United States. Ver Beck spent six months preparing for her book, interviewing many Freiburg mothers of several nationalities and translating almost 200,000 words in foreign medical reports on the method.[34]

One American physician borrowed her translation of Gauss' important 1906 publication describing the Twilight Sleep, an act that suggests some American physicians did not strictly adhere to the method because they had not read an accurate account of it.[35] Believing that power was inherent in knowledge and that women had to be able to argue "with authority," Ver Beck succeeded in making her book "technically irreproachable."[36] Other lay advocates also based their written work on extensive literature reviews as well as on interviews with physicians and Twilight Sleep mothers.

Few physicians who wrote on the subject of the Twilight Sleep, in particular, or on pain relief in childbirth, in general, failed to notice the antagonistic nature of the debate and the threat it posed to their claims of medical expertise. Physicians prior to 1914 had argued among themselves about the Twilight Sleep. But after the appearance of the *McClure's* article, as well as other newspaper and magazine features, they were forced to argue with very knowledgeable women and compelled to defend themselves against charges in the popular press that they had failed to execute their professional obligations in the matter of pain relief for women in childbirth. Both professional and popular literature carried a rather steady stream of charges and countercharges concerning the Twilight Sleep.

On the one side, lay activists and the physicians who supported them congratulated women for having brought the Twilight Sleep to the attention of the American public, thereby creating a demand for it that, in turn, forced physicians to reexamine the method and improve their skill in providing it. On the other side, the majority of physicians who were writers denounced the quackery, commercialism, and German origins of the Twilight Sleep as well as the lay intrusion into the domain of medicine.[37] Insisting that the German "masters" did not "own" the method and that they had tried it in good conscience and found it wanting, American physicians accused Gauss and Kronig of propagandizing the Twilight Sleep for their own benefit.[38] They also accused those women who praised the Germans for having given women the "third great

tenderness" and who bore their children in Germany of engendering disloyalty to the United States.[39]

While the Twilight Sleep debate revealed the rather tenuous relationship between medical experts and the public they
sought to serve, it also emphasized the importance of "science" in solving problems. Like other reform efforts of the time,
the Twilight Sleep movement was based on the premise that
progress in any area and the solution to any problem lay in
science.[40] Although it neither originated from scientific inves-
tigation nor utilized scientific methodology, the Twilight Sleep
was promoted as the scientific solution to the problem of pain
in labor. Since Twilight Sleep advocates believed that pain was
the cause of most complications in labor, the Twilight Sleep
was also promoted as the scientific solution to the greater
problem of childbirth itself. The Twilight Sleep not only made
childbirth safer and natural again, thus solving the problem
of high maternal and infant mortality and morbidity, but it
also made women less reluctant to have children. Accordingly,
the method was also viewed as a solution to the problem of
the declining birth rate among the upper classes.[41]

Despite women's successful agitation for the method, the
problems long associated with the Twilight Sleep continued to
surface. Some of these problems were inherent in the method
itself. Even under the best of circumstances, the Twilight Sleep
caused such complications as delayed labor and infant respiratory depression, which required intervention with other drugs
and instruments. Moreover, the Twilight Sleep was only appropriate for certain women. For example, even such strict
adherents to the Freiburg technique as James A. Harrar and
Ross McPherson, physicians who readopted the method after
having abandoned it, noted the slow advance of the fetal head
to the pelvic outlet in the second stage of labor, which required the application of forceps or the administration of Pi-
tuitrin, a drug used to augment uterine contractions.

They also reported having found it necessary to select those
women who would receive the treatment. Women in early labor or very active labor were not good candidates for the Twilight Sleep because it would stop the labor in the first in-

stance and be ineffective against pain in the second. Of the
one hundred women Harrar and McPherson studied who had
received the treatment, twenty had not responded to it at all
and were conscious of pain throughout their labors. Moreover,
these physicians indicated that "it requires the nicest judgment to suit the [memory] test to the standard of the intelligence of a given case, especially in patients of the lower grades
of mentality."[42]

German physicians themselves reported that the Twilight
Sleep sometimes caused delayed labor and neonatal apnea and
listed the contraindications of the method in certain women.[43]
In short, while skilled attendants were able to reduce the incidence of complications by carefully screening patients before
administering the treatment and by carefully attending women
under the influence of the treatment, the interaction of the
drugs with both a phenomenon as unpredictable as labor and
with the individual personality variables in laboring women
limited the extent to which they could achieve such a goal. In
fact, efforts to standardize the Twilight Sleep so that it could
be easily used by any physician on any patient anywhere failed
as physicians recognized the difficulty of standardizing the
management of a natural phenomenon such as labor.[44]

There were also a number of problems external to the Twilight Sleep but inherent in American obstetric care. For example, one physician noted that there were no physicians
trained as "Gausses" and "Kronigs" in the United States; there
were no obstetric residents and midwives trained to provide
the kind of skilled obstetric care required by the Twilight Sleep;
and American hospitals were located, in direct contrast to the
Freiburg clinic, on noisy streets, which detracted from the potential success of the method. He also indicated that general
practitioners were just too busy to provide the Twilight Sleep.[45]

Other reports concerning the difficulty of incorporating the
Twilight Sleep into American obstetric practice revealed that
the hospital was preferable to the home in providing the
treatment, but, since most women still labored in the home and
many with midwives, the treatment was offered at home or
ruled out for many women.[46] Furthermore, the serious demand for the Twilight Sleep forced physicians who were not

expert in the treatment, but who depended on obstetric patients for a significant portion of their incomes, to employ the method with potentially disastrous results. There are indications that general practitioners did in fact use the method improperly after 1915, sometimes for the purpose of maintaining a competitive edge over obstetric specialists who were attracting patients and higher fees by offering the treatment.[47]

Twilight Sleep enthusiasm waned with the recognition of the problems attending the method. Moreover, the death in 1915 of a noted advocate of the Twilight Sleep—a death wrongfully attributed to the method—also served to cool the furor.[48] Yet, while the Twilight Sleep movement itself lost momentum, it had, nevertheless, irrevocably altered the approach to the problem of pain relief in labor.

First, the agitation for the Twilight Sleep had "reawakened in the medical profession an acute interest"[49] in pain relief in labor and had made pain relief "the chief problem of the average physician who practices obstetrics."[50] The physician could no longer ignore the pain of childbirth by attributing it to natural law or divine will.

Second, the Twilight Sleep introduced the possibility that pain relief in labor could be safely and effectively achieved over the entire labor period, not just during the delivery phase. Significantly, while both physicians and women expected pain to accompany labor, they no longer accepted it as inevitable. By emphasizing the hazards of experiencing pain in childbirth and the benefits of pain relief, professional and lay advocates of the Twilight Sleep successfully convinced physicians that although pain relief in labor was difficult to achieve, it was still a legitimate and even necessary goal toward which they should strive. Few physicians after 1915 believed that it was wrong or unwise to attempt to provide pain relief, even in normal labors.

Third, the successful use of a drug regimen by a number of physicians and women's positive responses to it served to direct physicians' efforts toward finding the drug regimen most suitable for labor. While physicians recognized the importance of psychological factors, such as fear, in the pain experience, they saw drugs, not a method that was itself psychological, as the best measure against pain in labor. Despite all of the uncertainties of drug use, after 1915, pain relief in labor, with few exceptions, implied the use of drugs.

The Twilight Sleep movement also contributed to an important change in the conduct of American childbirth. First, the Twilight Sleep further justified the presence of the male physician in the lying-in chamber. The very nature of the method, namely, a drug regimen, ruled out the midwife or any non-physician who generally did not use drugs or instruments as the source of the treatment. Although women advocates of the Twilight Sleep were very angry with physicians for not providing them with the treatment sooner, they, nevertheless, turned to physicians, courted them, and pressured them to adopt a method over which only a physician could have ultimate control. Women themselves helped physicians replace midwives as chief birth attendants and helped them become the dominant figures in maternity care.

Second, the Twilight Sleep was a key factor in legitimating the transfer of birth from the home to the hospital. While some physicians maintained that the treatment could be safely administered in the home, the majority insisted that if women wanted pain relief over the entire labor period, they would have to go to the hospital to obtain it. Not only did the hospital, according to these physicians, house the trained attendants and the equipment required to provide a safe and effective Twilight Sleep birth in a convenient manner, but it also prevented the family and friends of the laboring woman from intruding on the sensory isolation required by the method. Moreover, the hospital allowed easy access to the instruments that were often required to offset the complications induced by the method.

Third, the Twilight Sleep focused both professional and public attention on the complexity and potential hazards of childbirth and on the need for trained and vigilant specialists to manage it. After 1915, childbirth was increasingly viewed as a condition, the most important symptom of which, pain, needed to be treated to prevent injury and death. In addition, obstetrics was increasingly depicted as a surgical specialty that warranted the incorporation of the anesthesia, antisepsis, and instrumental intervention characterizing surgery. Most importantly, since Twilight Sleep advocates believed that the method made modern childbirth natural again, unassisted childbirth was, by default, unnatural. By altering the conceptualization of *natural* and *artificial*, as these terms related to the process of birth, the Twilight Sleep contributed to a change in the philosophical foundation upon which the practice of obstetrics was based.

The Twilight Sleep movement also revealed some interesting ambiguities or contradictions in the arguments of some women advocates of the method. These women believed that the emancipation of women depended, in part, on women's liberation from their biological functions. Eager to escape what they perceived as the horrors of childbirth, they apparently saw no contradiction in seeking influence in society by surrendering their control over their mental and bodily functions in childbirth to others. Moreover, while eager to demonstrate that women were equal to men, they emphasized how unequal women and men were in terms of the burdens their biological functions placed on them. If these women intended to argue their way out of the limited sphere in which women were placed by virtue of their unique biological functions, they ultimately succeeded in arguing their way back into it by acknowledging the extent to which maternity ruled a woman's body and mind. The Twilight Sleep reinforced the idea that maternity was a woman's most important task but that it made women more prone to physical and mental illness. Moreover, it accentuated the idea that women needed special help and protection by virtue of their ability to give birth.[51]

The Twilight Sleep movement also illustrated how important the popular press and public demand were in changing obstetric practice. Because of the physician's already tenuous position as attendant to the childbearing woman, in part, because of moral objections to male involvement in an intimate female function and, in part, because of charges of "meddlesome midwifery," obstetrics was much more subject to public pressure than other medical specialties.[52] While few individuals to this date challenge the surgeon's expertise in or right to perform surgery, for example, a segment of the public has

always challenged both the expertise of the physician in obstetrics and his right to practice it at all in normal cases (the
major portion of obstetric practice). While physicians bitterly
resented public pressure to alter their practice in the case of
the Twilight Sleep, they also learned the value of courting the
media and the public to gather support for themselves. Indeed, by the end of the 1930s, physicians who attended childbearing women had learned how to use the press to convert
popular demand to professional gain. The Twilight Sleep furor was a most important lesson for them.

In summary, women's agitation for the Twilight Sleep
strengthened the idea that pain best defined childbirth, that
pain was to be avoided, and that pain relief was to be sought.
Yet, while the Twilight Sleep allowed women some control over
physicians and the way childbirth was conducted, the net effect of the debate was a transfer of control to physicians in the
management of childbirth.[53] Understandably viewing childbirth as synonymous with suffering and death, both women
and physicians agreed that whether life or death awaited the
woman in childbirth, she was better off unconscious. If she
awakened from childbirth uninjured, so much the better. If she
never awakened, what had she really lost?

Notes

1. Marguerite Tracy and Constance Leupp, "Painless Childbirth," *McClure's*, June 1914, pp. 37–51. On the response this article
evoked see William Armstrong, "The 'Twilight Sleep' at Freiburg,"
Woman's Home Companion, September 1914, pp. 4, 69; Mary Boyd
and Marguerite Tracy, "More About Painless Childbirth," *McClure's*,
October 1914, pp. 56–59; Alice Hamilton, "Dammerschlaf," *Survey*,
7 November 1914, pp. 158–59; and "Is the Twilight Sleep Safe—For
Me?" *Woman's Home Companion*, January 1915, pp. 10, 43.

2. Boyd and Tracy, "More About Painless Childbirth," p. 63.

3. Hanna Rion Ver Beck, *The Truth About Twilight Sleep* (New
York: McBride, Nast, 1915), foreword and p. 359.

4. Ibid., p. 1.

5. Mary Boyd, "The Story of Dammerschlaf," *Survey*, 7 November
1914, pp. 125–29.

6. James Young Simpson quoted by Marguerite Tracy and Mary

Boyd in *Painless Childbirth* (New York: Frederick A. Stokes, 1915), p. xxx.

7. Ibid., p. 41.

8. John Duffy, "Anglo-American Reaction to Obstetrical Anesthesia," *Bulletin of the History of Medicine* 38 (January-February 1964):32–33; Palmer Findley, *Priests of Lucina: The Story of Obstetrics* (Boston: Little, Brown, 1939), pp. 236–38; Roy P. Finney, *The Story of Motherhood* (New York: Liveright, 1937), pp. 156–60; Alan Frank Guttmacher, *Into This Universe: The Story of Human Birth* (New York: Viking Press, 1937), pp. 196–97; Howard W. Haggard, *Devils, Drugs, and Doctors: The Story of the Science of Healing From Medicine-Man to Doctor* (New York: Harper and Brothers, 1929), pp. 93–97; Claude Edwin Heaton, "The History of Anesthesia and Analgesia in Obstetrics," *Journal of the History of Medicine and Allied Sciences* 1 (October 1946):567; M. Pierce Rucker, "An Eighteenth Century Method of Pain Relief in Obstetrics," *Journal of the History of Medicine and Allied Sciences* 5 (Winter 1950):101–5; and A. Clair Siddall, "Bloodletting in American Obstetric Practice, 1800–1945," *Bulletin of the History of Medicine* 54 (Spring 1980):101–10.

9. Duffy, "Anglo-American Reactions," pp. 33–42; Heaton, "History of Anesthesia," pp. 570–71.

10. Duffy, "Anglo-American Reactions," pp. 33–35.

11. Martin Steven Pernick, "A Calculus of Suffering: Pain, Anesthesia, and Utilitarian Professionalism in Nineteenth Century American Medicine" (Ph.D. dissertation, Columbia University, 1979), pp. 84–85, 345.

12. Ibid., pp. 54–127.

13. Walter Channing, *A Treatise on Etherization in Childbirth* (Boston: William D. Ticknor, 1848), pp. 135–58; Duffy, "Anglo-American Reaction," pp. 35–42.

14. Pernick, "A Calculus of Suffering," pp. 271–366.

15. Jane B. Donegan, *Women and Men Midwives: Medicine, Morality, and Misogyny in Early America* (Westport, Conn.: Greenwood Press, 1978); Judy Barrett Litoff, *American Midwives: 1860 to the Present* (Westport, Conn.: Greenwood Press, 1978); and Catherine M. Scholten, " 'On the Importance of the Obstetrick Art': Changing Customs of Childbirth in America, 1760–1825," *William and Mary Quarterly* 34 (July 1977):426–45. Recent scholarship on childbirth suggests that women turned away from midwives and toward physicians for the relief from suffering physicians offered them and that midwives were either prevented from learning how to use instruments or preferred not using any artificial measures in childbirth.

16. "Anesthesia in Midwifery," *Boston Medical and Surgical Jour-*

nal, 9 December 1858, pp. 369–73; Duffy, "Anglo-American Reactions," p. 38; Haggard, *Devils, Drugs, and Doctors*, pp. 120–21; and Harold Speert, *The Sloane Hospital Chronicle* (Philadelphia: F. A. Davis, 1963), p. 227.

17. Grace L. Meigs, *Maternal Mortality From All Conditions Connected with Childbirth in the United States and Certain Other Countries*, U.S. Children's Bureau Pub. 19 (Washington, D.C.: Government Printing Office, 1917).

18. G. J. Barker-Benfield, *The Horrors of the Half-Known Life: Male Attitudes Toward Women and Sexuality in Nineteenth-Century America* (New York: Harper Colophon Books, 1977); Donegan, *Women and Men Midwives*; Barbara Ehrenreich and Deirdre English, *For Her Own Good: 150 Years of the Experts' Advice to Women* (Garden City, N.Y.: Anchor Press/Doubleday, 1978); John S. Haller and Robin M. Haller, *The Physician and Sexuality in Victorian America* (New York: W. W. Norton, 1977); Litoff, *American Midwives*; Scholten "On the Importance of the Obstetrick Art"; Sarah Stage, *Female Complaints: Lydia Pinkham and the Business of Women's Medicine* (New York: W. W. Norton, 1979); and Richard W. Wertz and Dorothy C. Wertz, *Lying-In: A History of Childbirth in America* (New York: Free Press, 1977).

19. Carl Henry Davis, *Painless Childbirth Eutocia and Nitrous Oxid-Oxygen Analgesia* (Chicago: Forbes, 1916), p. 13.

20. Ibid., p. 18.

21. Charlotte Teller, "The Neglected Psychology of the 'Twilight Sleep,'" *Good Housekeeping*, July 1915, pp. 17–24.

22. Bertha Van Hoosen, *Scopolamine-Morphine Anesthesia* (Chicago: House of Manz, 1915), p. 101.

23. Ibid., p. 90.

24. Woodbridge Hall Birchmore, "The Hyoscine Sleep in Obstetric Practice," *Medical Record*, 12 January 1907, pp. 58–60.

25. The description that follows is primarily from James A. Harrar and Ross McPherson, "Scopolamine-Narcophin Seminarcosis in Labor," *Bulletin of the Lying-In Hospital of the City of New York* 10 (February 1915):40–48. These physicians were strict adherents of the German technique.

26. Ibid., p. 45.

27. "Accusing the Medical Profession," *New York Times*, 17 September 1914, p. 8; Samuel Wyllis Bandler, *The Expectant Mother* (Philadelphia: W. B. Saunders, 1916), p. 144; "Enthusiasm Carried to Excess," *New York Times*, 12 February 1915, p. 10; Harrar and McPherson, "Scopolamine-Narcophin," p. 42; William H. Wellington Knipe, "'The Twilight Sleep' From the Hospital Viewpoint," *Modern*

Hospital 3 (October 1914):250; H. W. Kostmayer, "A Practical Method of Minimizing the Pain of Labor," *New Orleans Medical and Surgical Journal* 69 (July 1916):88–90; E. M. Lazard, "The Twilight Sleep Propaganda in the Lay Press," *Southern California Practitioner* 30 (January 1915): 17; and W. R. Livingston, "Deductions From Experience With 'Twilight Sleep' at St. John's Hospital, Oxnard," *Southern California Practitioner* 30 (July 1915):221.

28. There were arguments about whether narcophin or morphine and scopolamine or hyoscine were better. These arguments reflected competition between American and German pharmaceutical houses and among American houses. See Russell Kelso Carter, *The Sleeping Car 'Twilight' or Motherhood Without Pain* (Boston: Chapple Publishing, 1915), and Livingston, "Deductions from Experience," p. 222.

29. Carter, "Sleeping Car," p. 174. See also Ver Beck, "Truth About Twilight Sleep," p. 26.

30. Teller, "Neglected Psychology," pp. 20–21.

31. Boyd and Tracy, "More About Painless Childbirth," p. 110.

32. Ibid., p. xxxiii.

33. Ibid.

34. Ver Beck, foreword and pp. 26–33.

35. Ibid., p. 328. According to her, there was no published translation of Gauss' work available in the United States.

36. Ibid., p. 63.

37. "A Story of 'Ethics' Violated," *New York Times*, 5 February 1915, p. 10; "Deny Insanity is Due to 'Twilight Sleep,' " *New York Times*, 7 November 1914, p. 7; William Gillespie, "Analgesics and Anesthetics in Labor: Their Indications and Contraindications," *Ohio State Medical Journal* 11 (October 1915):612; A. L. Mann, "Is Twilight Sleep to be 'For Me.' A Blessing—Or a Curse?" *Illinois Medical Journal* 27 (April 1915):264–69; "The 'Twilight Sleep' Again," *Literary Digest*, 15 August 1914, p. 265; "The 'Twilight Sleep' Dispute," *Literary Digest*, 19 September 1914, p. 506; " 'Twilight Sleep' and Medical Publicity," *Literary Digest*, 11 July 1914, pp. 60–61; and "Spoiling a Frank Admission," *New York Times*, 5 April 1915, p. 10.

38. "Is the Twilight Sleep Safe—For Me?" *Woman's Home Companion*, p. 42. Some physicians maintained that the Twilight Sleep was like the American physician George Crile's "anociassociation" method for surgery. See " 'Twilight Sleep' is Successful in 120 Cases Here," *New York Times*, 30 August 1914, sec. 4, p. 8.

39. According to " 'Twilight Sleep,' " *Nation,* 12 August 1915, p. 211, the first two "tendernesses" were the introduction of chloroform into obstetric practice and American gynecological surgery.

40. For the emergence of "science" as a key factor in American thought, see Richard Hofstadter, *Social Darwinism in American Thought* (Boston: Beacon Press, 1955); Charles Rosenberg, *No Other Gods: On Science and American Social Thought* (Baltimore: Johns Hopkins University Press, 1976); and Robert Wiebe, *The Search For Order, 1877–1920* (New York: Hill and Wang, 1967), pp. 133–63.

41. Although the Twilight Sleep debate does not appear in accounts of American eugenic thought known to the author, advocates of the method and, indeed, of pain-relieving measures throughout the first half of the twentieth century appear to have been informed by what Kenneth M. Ludmerer, in *Genetics and American Society: A Historical Appraisal* (Baltimore: Johns Hopkins University Press, 1972), described as "positive eugenics," or the desire to encourage the reproduction of those individuals considered most "fit." While Twilight Sleep advocates saw the method as appropriate for *all* women, they believed that it was *necessary* for the favored woman to survive childbirth. This was in line with the belief that the lower classes of women felt very little pain and, therefore, had few problems in labor. This was clearly not the case, but the Twilight Sleep should not be viewed as a "negative eugenic" (racist or classist) effort per se since it did not have as its primary goal the prevention of the "unfit" from reproducing. Moreover, Twilight Sleep advocates believed that healthier babies would be born also. For other references on American eugenic thought, see Linda Gordon, *Woman's Body, Woman's Right: A Social History of Birth Control in America* (New York: Grossman, Penguin Books, 1977), pp. 116–58; Mark H. Haller, *Eugenics: Hereditarian Attitudes in American Thought* (New Brunswick, N.J.: Rutgers University Press, 1963); and Donald K. Pickens, *Eugenics and the Progressives* (Nashville, Tenn.: Vanderbilt University Press, 1968). This line of thinking was suggested to the author by Dr. Darwin Stapleton.

42. Harrar and McPherson, "Scopolamine-Narcophin," pp. 43–47.

43. Mann, "Is Twilight Sleep," p. 266; Geheinroth Professor Dr. Kronig, "The Difference Between the Older and Newer Treatments by X-Ray and Radium in Gynecological Diseases," *Surgery, Gynecology and Obstetrics* 18 (May 1914):529–32. Kronig digressed from the title subject to a discussion of the Twilight Sleep.

44. Examples of such efforts were the Siegel method and the H-M-C tablet (hyoscine, morphine, and cactin).

45. Alfred M. Hellman, *Amnesia and Analgesia in Parturition* (New York: Paul B. Hoeber, 1915), pp. 105, 158.

46. Knipe, " 'Twilight Sleep' From the Hospital Viewpoint," pp. 250–51.

47. R. L. Raiford, "Painless Labor," *Virginia Medical Monthly* 51 (June 1923):152–55. In general, obstetricians were worried about general practitioners, with whom they were in competition for patients, adopting techniques they were unskilled to perform. For general practitioners, obstetric patients were important as an entrée into the family for other medical needs. In addition, some women were so adamant about receiving the treatment that they suggested bringing lawsuits against physicians for "negligent malpractice" if they did not offer it. See " 'Twilight Sleep,' " *New York Times*, 11 February 1915, p. 8.

48. "Doctors Disagree on Twilight Sleep," *New York Times*, 24 August 1915, p. 7; "Mrs. Francis X. Carmody Buried," *New York Times*, 25 August 1915, p. 11; and "To Fight Twilight Sleep," *New York Times*, 31 August 1915, p. 5.

49. Hellman, *Amnesia and Analgesia*, pp. 8–9.

50. Davis, *Painless Childbirth*, p. 27.

51. The Twilight Sleep debate underscored women's growing visibility outside the home. The foremost champions of the method were also activists for other women's issues such as suffrage, birth control, and improved factory conditions for women and children. Clubwomen, women professionals, reformers, and feminists of all persuasions made up the movement. While they may have diverged on many women's issues, they generally agreed that women's greatest source of influence derived from motherhood. Jill Conway, in "Women Reformers and American Culture, 1870–1930," *Journal of Social History* 5 (Winter 1971–72):164–77, noted that support of birth control or divorce, for example, which on the surface appears to challenge the family and motherhood, was not incompatible with the idealization of the family and motherhood. In the same vein, emphasizing the horrors of childbirth is not necessarily rejecting maternity. Yet, as June Sochen, in *Movers and Shakers: American Women Thinkers and Activists, 1900–1970* (New York: Quadrangle/New York Times Book, 1973), pp. 1–30, suggested, if women concede anything to *nature*, their arguments for equality with men are vulnerable. Accordingly, the Twilight Sleep advocacy can be viewed as supporting a feminist or antifeminist position. See also, in regard to the Twilight Sleep as a women's issue, Judith Walzer Leavitt, "Birthing and Anesthesia: The Debate Over Twilight Sleep," *Signs: Journal of Women in Culture and Society* 6 (Autumn 1980):147–65 and Laurence G. Miller, "Pain, Parturition, and the Profession: Twilight Sleep

in America," in *Health Care in America: Essays in Social History*, ed. Susan Reverby and David Rosner (Philadelphia: Temple University Press, 1979), pp. 19–44.

52. Wertz and Wertz, *Lying-In*.

53. Leavitt, "Birthing and Anesthesia."

2 ———

THE CONQUEST OF PAIN: UNDER THE INFLUENCE OF DRUGS ————

Between the summer of 1915, when the Twilight Sleep furor was ending, and the fall of 1948, when the Natural Childbirth craze was beginning, the most significant event relative to the problem of pain relief in childbirth was the extensive use in labor and delivery of virtually every drug known to be effective in producing analgesia, amnesia, and anesthesia in human beings suffering from pain. During this period, physicians and, to a lesser extent, nurses published descriptions of the uses, methods and routes of administration, and benefits and liabilities of an almost staggering array of drugs for pain relief in labor. These included narcotic and nonnarcotic analgesics, barbiturates and other sedative, hypnotic, and tranquilizing drugs as well as chemical agents for local, regional, and general anesthesia.

A woman laboring in her home prior to 1915 might have received ether, chloroform, or nitrous oxide and oxygen by inhalation to relieve her of pain in the second stage of labor (the delivery period). By 1948, it was more likely that a woman laboring in the hospital would receive one or a combination of pharmacologic agents orally, rectally, hypodermically, by inhalation, or by direct infiltration of the nervous pathways to the uterus, cervix, or perineum as early as the first stage of labor and frequently before the cervix was dilated to five centimeters.

While medical practitioners formerly viewed the use of drugs for pain relief in childbirth as an option generally restricted to the most active parts of labor or for women in unusual circumstances, after the Twilight Sleep debate of 1914–1915, it increasingly became the *duty* of the physician to provide pain relief for as much of the labor as was possible within the limits of safety. It was as well the *right* of the woman to demand it.[1] Arthur Bill, a prominent Cleveland obstetrician, remarked in 1932 that the "principle of the relief of pain [in childbirth] is almost universally accepted."[2] By 1941, "analgesia to the point of amnesia" was virtually routine in the majority of large hospitals.[3]

Indeed, by the end of the 1940s, virtually every physician who wrote on the subject of pain relief in childbirth believed that it was the moral and professional obligation of all physicians to relieve pain, and many commented that the Twilight Sleep debate had awakened everyone to the possibility that labor pain could be relieved. Moreover, like Twilight Sleep advocates, physicians tied pain relief in labor to the emancipation of women and to the advancement of both civilization and the profession of obstetrics.[4] Most importantly, for physicians, pain relief in labor meant the use of drugs.

Yet exercising this professional obligation was no simple matter for either the physician who prescribed drugs for the treatment of pain in labor or for the nurse who generally administered them and supervised the patient afterward. The alleviation of pain in labor with drugs presented professionals with a number of safety problems that their counterparts in surgery did not have to face. James Young Simpson's remark that "the application of anesthesia to midwifery involves many more difficult and delicate problems than its mere application to surgery" suggests that nineteenth-century physicians recognized the complications resulting from drug use in childbirth, even if they lacked accurate knowledge of the specific physiological events involved.[5] For example, physicians had always noticed the problems of delayed labor and neonatal respiratory depression.[6]

Four major problems distinctively attended drug use in labor.[7] First, virtually every drug given to the laboring woman also passed to the fetus through the placenta or indirectly affected the fetus by altering a key function in the mother, such as the oxygenation of her blood or the maintenance of her blood pressure. Accordingly, professional attendants had to account for the action and potential side and toxic effects of every drug they selected and administered in both the laboring woman and the fetus. Unlike the surgeon or surgical nurse, the physician and nurse who attended the woman in labor were responsible *at the same time* for two individuals with markedly dissimilar tolerance levels to drugs.

Second, unlike most surgical cases that were scheduled in advance, virtually all cases of labor, with the exception of elective inductions and cesarean sections, were *emergencies* in terms of the use of pain-relieving drugs. That is, professional attendants could elaborately prepare a surgical patient well in advance of the operation for the drugs he or she would receive in surgery. (This involved keeping the stomach empty and giving appropriate preanesthetic drugs to sedate the patient and to dry respiratory secretions. These preparations prevented the frequently fatal aspiration of stomach contents into the lungs during surgery and permitted easier and safer induction of anesthesia.) In contrast, no professional could guarantee exactly when a woman would start her labor.

Third, certain features of maternal physiology, such as delayed emptying of the stomach and the imposition of the enlarged and heavy uterus on respiratory muscles and major blood vessels, made the administration of drugs an extremely hazardous undertaking. In the case of delayed emptying of the stomach, even if a woman had not eaten for several hours prior to the onset of labor, there was no guarantee that her stomach would be empty by the time she received general anesthesia at the beginning of the second stage of labor.

Fourth, while the average operation might last up to four hours, a labor might last up to twenty hours, requiring the use of a greater variety of drugs and methods or greater cumulative doses of drugs for effective pain relief. In addition to this, many drugs used for pain relief in labor and delivery directly altered the functioning of the muscles of the uterus, either during the labor itself or after delivery. A narcotic analgesic,

such as morphine, could either shorten the duration of a labor
by facilitating cervical dilatation, or it could lengthen the
duration of labor by stopping uterine contractions altogether,
depending on when in the labor it was given. Gaseous anesthetics given in the second stage might facilitate the delivery
by relaxing uterine muscles and contribute to a maternal
hemorrhage after delivery because of the same effect.

Consequently, professionals had to predict on the basis of
their knowledge of the average duration of a *natural* labor (that
is, without artificial interference of any kind) in both primiparas (women having their first babies) and multiparas (with
generally shorter labors than primiparas) when it was best to
give a certain drug. They constantly faced the questions, when
was it too soon or too late, in terms of the action of the uterine
muscles in labor, to give a drug? If it was appropriate to give
a drug at a certain time in the labor in terms of the uterine
muscles, was it inappropriate to give the drug at that time in
terms of the safety of the infant? Most drugs given for pain
relief in the first stage of labor were dangerous for the infant
if administered within two to four hours of the expected time
of delivery since the infant would have to initiate respirations
on his own at the moment when these drugs reached their peak
effect in the body. Unlike surgical attendants, professionals
attending the woman in labor had to contend with a phenomenon that in its natural state was often unpredictable in terms
of time of onset and duration.

In short, the safe and effective use of pain-relieving drugs
in childbirth demanded a breadth and depth of knowledge in
fetal and maternal physiology and pharmacology that average
professional practitioners often did not have and that they could
not have had given the state of knowledge about the fetus and
neonate at the time. Moreover, professionals needed a preci-
sion in timing and forecasting not demanded of the physician
or nurse who administered these drugs to one *prepared* surgical patient at a time for a relatively brief and usually *predictable* period of time. Furthermore, once a woman received
the first dose of a drug in labor, her attendants' prediction about
the likely duration of her labor, founded as it was on their understanding of the average length of labor in the natural state,

was no longer valid if the drug served to speed the labor up or slow it down. Accordingly, as professionals began to rely on pain-relieving drugs in labor, the knowledge they already possessed about the characteristics of natural labor became correspondingly less useful to them.

Indeed, professionals indicated that patient behavior, normally the most useful criterion for evaluating the progress of labor, was rendered unreliable because of the effects of these drugs.[8] Without performing frequent vaginal or rectal examinations, which predisposed women to infection (a dreaded consequence prior to the widespread use of antibiotics after World War II), the experienced caregiver could determine the progress of labor by such behavioral signposts as a woman's awareness of her surroundings, her willingness to talk to her attendants, her moans, and her desire to bear down. Yet, under the influence of pain-relieving drugs, women no longer manifested the behavior that correlated so well with the physiological course of labor. Those women who received amnesic drugs slept throughout their labors, were continually restless, agitated, or crying, thrashed about with contractions and slept soundly between them; or, if they were apparently awake were totally unconscious of what was happening to them. Those women who received regional block anesthesia lost sensation in the lower half of their bodies, and, even though awake and aware, they were also unable to determine when their "time" had arrived.

Consequently, physicians and nurses were forced to resort to more intrusive means to determine labor progress. They were compelled to look at a woman's genitals more often, if only to assure themselves that the infant had not been born without their knowledge. They were forced to perform more rectal and vaginal examinations to determine the condition of the cervix and the descent of the fetus. They were compelled to palpate her abdomen more often to determine the characteristics of her contractions.[9]

Most importantly, the use of pain-relieving drugs in labor made professionals view their patients as less helpful to them in guiding their actions than they used to be. In fact, the use of these drugs made women definitely "uncooperative." Vir-

tually all of the pain-relieving regimens used in the first stage
of labor between 1915 and 1948, with the exception of regional block anesthesia, tended to cause excitement, restless-
ness, confusion, delirium, and even "frenzy" in the patient.[10]
Primarily designed to produce analgesia (pain relief) by in-
ducing amnesia, these regimens did not block women's sensation of pain but rather distorted their consciousness of it.
Consequently, the laboring woman under the influence of drugs
such as scopolamine, paraldehyde, and nembutal could be
verbally and physically abusive to herself or to her attendants
in her efforts to seek relief from the pain she was still experiencing. Professionals emphasized the importance of uninter-
rupted supervision by trained attendants of women receiving
these drugs as well as the use of measures such as restraints
and padded cribs to protect them from harm.[11] They also noted
that it was sometimes necessary to use *additional pain-relieving
drugs* during the delivery to maintain aseptic conditions, since
unruly patients grabbed at their specially cleansed genitals and
the sterile drapes covering them.[12]

Despite their realization that providing pain relief in labor
was often more complex than the problem of pain itself, and
despite their growing understanding of the many undesirable
effects of these drugs, professionals, especially physicians, after
1915, increasingly viewed the use of these drugs as the sine
qua non of *any* (normal or operative) well-managed and properly conducted labor. For example, Joseph B. DeLee, one of the
two obstetrical "titans"[13] of the early twentieth century, had
noted in the second edition of his book, *The Principles and
Practice of Obstetrics*, published in 1915, that his experiences
with the use of pain-relieving drugs in the first stage of labor
had led him to dispense with their use completely during this
period, except in unusual circumstances.[14] But, by 1920, in the
third edition of his text, he indicated that it was the "duty" of
the physician to relieve women of labor pain and included more
information on the use of nitrous oxide with oxygen—an anesthetic that could be used at the end of the first stage of labor.[15] In the 1925 edition of his work, he stated that he "usually" gave morphine and scopolamine during the first stage of
labor and, sometimes, heroin.[16] By 1929, in his fifth edition,

he described even more drugs and drug regimens for use in all stages of labor.[17]

The other obstetrical titan of the period, J. Whitridge Williams, also demonstrated the gradual acceptance of pain-relieving drugs as appropriate for the entire labor period in successive editions of his text.[18] Arthur Bill, a strong advocate of pharmacologic pain relief, stated in 1922 that even those physicians most strongly opposed to the use of obstetric anesthesia and analgesia were now in favor of their use.[19] He re-emphasized in 1937 that despite some renewed medical opposition to the use of these drugs in labor, the real question of the day was not whether to make labor painless but rather how to do it in the best way.[20]

Many physicians were initially reluctant to employ pain-relieving drugs routinely in labor, and some were never enthusiastic about them, but they still increasingly used them for two major reasons. First, in their view, women were forcing them to do so.[21] One Southern physician asserted that women had forced physicians to adopt an "up and doing" stance in obstetric work. Moreover, the physician who refused to give women what they wanted would soon become unpopular with them.[22]

Second, physicians thought that modern obstetric practice demanded the use of drugs.[23] Although physicians believed that women's demands were compelling them to use drugs, often against their better judgment, they also suggested that their own desires to make obstetrics as modern, scientific, and prestigious a specialty as surgery warranted the use of the latest techniques in the care of childbearing women. After the reintroduction of the Twilight Sleep into American obstetric practice, few issues in the medical care of the laboring woman provoked as much interest and experimentation as the use of these drugs. (One physician even noted that he had made a "hobby" of obstetric anesthesia and analgesia.)[24]

Moreover, physicians equated the use of drugs and instruments with progress toward the goal of scientific obstetric care. Consequently, any physician practicing obstetrics who was interested in pleasing his patients and committed to modernizing the specialty so that it would never again be confused with mere midwifery could hardly avoid using these drugs, no matter how reluctant he might have been to do so. The "twilight sleeping car" had gained momentum swiftly, and the physician who missed it also risked his reputation and practice.

Furthermore, as physicians became more accustomed to using these drugs throughout the labor period, they also became more accustomed to and more willing to accept some of the side effects of these drugs. For example, one of the reasons that the Twilight Sleep had lost favor in American physicians between 1906 and 1914 was the noticeable number of babies born with breathing difficulties.[25] Already somewhat reluctant to use pain-relieving drugs, particularly in the first stage of labor, physicians were alarmed by the specter of injured or dead babies caused by a medical regimen they were not convinced was necessary in the first place. But, by 1925, a medical advocate of pantopon-scopolamine seminarcosis in labor, one of many variations of the Twilight Sleep, suggested that temporary apnea, or delayed breathing, at birth might be advantageous to infants because they were less likely to aspirate amniotic fluid and, therefore, less likely to develop pulmonary complications— major causes of infant morbidity and mortality.[26]

Alan Guttmacher, a major figure in obstetrics, stated in 1937 that in practically all cases where the infant did not breathe at once, respirations started soon and the "permanent effect [of the delay] was greater on the obstetrician's nerves than on the baby."[27] A group of investigators reporting on their use of paraldehyde in labor and the opinions of their colleagues on the subject of neonatal apnea in 1940 confirmed that delayed respirations in infants at birth was an essentially harmless event.[28] And, Nicholson Eastman, another influential obstetrician, concluded that even though sedatives given in labor in amnesic doses inhibited the onset of respirations in 40 to 60 percent of cases, the administration of safe analgesia to women in labor at term was equivalent to offering no analgesia at all in terms of the "ultimate outcome."[29]

Indeed, by 1940, it was no longer clear that drugs used for pain relief in labor were *directly* responsible for infants' respiratory problems at birth. In their 1940 survey of fetal and neonatal death, Edith L. Potter and Fred L. Adair stated that "the importance of maternal anesthesia and analgesia in the production of cerebral injury in the fetus is extremely difficult to determine."[30] Allowing for the possibility that the infant's respiratory functions might be sufficiently depressed as a result of drug use in labor to cause death from oxygen deprivation, Potter and Adair concluded that "up to the present time there is no sufficiently well-controlled series of cases in which analgesics or anesthetics have been administered in a generally accepted manner to prove unequivocably that ill effects result directly from their use."[31]

Even if most physicians probably did not view temporary apnea in the infant as an advantage to be sought, they, as well as nurses, had become more skilled in resuscitating infants and had more equipment at their disposal to do so than their counterparts did twenty-five years before. As the use of pain-relieving drugs in labor became more extensive and routine, the temporary impairment of the infant's respiratory functions at birth was no longer so alarming to professionals as it had once been. Indeed, it was reasonable to expect it and prudent to anticipate it.

Physicians and nurses also increasingly anticipated problems concerning the laboring woman herself. For example, James A. Harrar, who changed his allegiance from the Twilight Sleep to the Gwathmey method of analgesia (rectal ether), noted the importance of adding quinine to the ether mixture to prevent delay in the second stage of labor.[32] Mary C. Blackwell, reviewing the nursing care of the obstetrical patient under the influence of drugs, indicated that a sufficient number of nurses could prevent the "well-managed" but confused patient from harming herself.[33] Other physicians suggested that the use of nitrous oxide and outlet forceps could offset the uncooperativeness of the patient who received amnesic drugs. The use of forceps, in particular, was really an advantage because it allowed the physician to control the delivery of the infant's head, thus preventing trauma to the fetus and the perineum.[34]

The liberal use of drugs was closely related to fundamental changes in obstetric goals, values, and practice. Over time, physicians and, to a lesser extent, nurses learned to anticipate and not to fear certain problems arising from the use of pain-relieving drugs in labor, and they also redefined some problems as advantages to be deliberately sought. Even more importantly, they learned to use pain-relieving drugs and instruments as preventive measures against these problems. Physicians converted some of the negative consequences of the *treatment* of pain in childbirth with drugs into positive ones with the *prophylactic* use of drugs and instruments.

An especially useful illustration of the gradual shift in reasoning behind the use of pain-relieving drugs from therapeutic to prophylactic is Howard F. Kane and George B. Roth's 1935 report on the use of paraldehyde in labor. These physicians stated that it was their "custom" to deliver by "outlet forceps practically all heads that reach the perineum" because they believed there was no value to the woman to have to bear down in the second stage of labor. Accordingly, they substituted the use of outlet forceps, which itself requires an episiotomy and anesthetic, for the woman's own efforts. Consequently, they were able to report that their use of paraldehyde in the first stage of labor did not lengthen the labor by interfering with a woman's ability to push and thus did not require increased operative intervention since they already used operative techniques to terminate labor in virtually 100 percent of their cases.[35]

Both the desire to protect the patient from the dangers of labor and to make it a more predictable and agreeable phenomenon infused the practice of the "new" obstetrics, which by the end of the 1930s was characterized by the routine prophylactic use of drugs and instruments. In fact, the increasing use of obstetric anesthesia and analgesia over the entire labor period after 1915 was viewed as the single most important factor contributing to the high incidence of operative intervention. This tendency to intervene was, in turn, viewed as the most distinctive feature of American obstetrics. Drugs not only necessitated more intervention, they also allowed more.

The Rise of Prophylactic Obstetrics

American physicians gradually developed a very ambivalent view of the natural process of birth. The extent to which this view derived from the suffering and death they witnessed in childbirth or from their need to define childbearing solely in terms of suffering and death is less clear. In any case, physician Austin Flint clearly conveyed this ambivalence in 1925 when he suggested that Americans should place more emphasis on the normality of childbirth and then stated that "under modern conditions, labor is not a normal function, and should not be so considered either by the profession or by the public."[36] Condemning both midwives and general practitioners for their lack of obstetric skills, Flint asked whether something that killed, injured, and caused pain and invalidism could be called normal.

Idealizing woman's natural function of maternity—but emphasizing how capricious and even lethal nature could be if left to "her" own devices in the lying-in chamber as well as the ineffectiveness of the modern woman in coping with natural labor—physicians successfully convinced the American public by the end of the 1930s how superior obstetrics was to midwifery. Obstetricians, in particular, underscored their separation from the midwife and from the general practitioner by pointing to the specialist's exclusive or greater judgment and skill in employing scientific advances (drugs and instruments) to defeat nature or, at least, to control her on the childbearing woman's behalf. As one physician put it, "nature no longer dominates the practice of obstetrics," and the obstetrician no longer "awaits her pleasure."[37]

The value of natural birth became increasingly suspect when the creation of the first birth registration area in 1915 made possible the publication of the first reliable maternal and infant mortality statistics.[38] While women certainly knew of injury and death in childbirth from personal experience, Americans now read about the extraordinarily high mortality associated with maternity in the United States.

In the first three and one-half decades of the twentieth century, deaths associated with maternity were commonplace. George Clark Mosher reported in 1924 that there were 16,000 maternity-related deaths each year over the previous twenty years.[39] In 1915, 61 women died per 10,000 live births. The death rate rose to 92 per 10,000 live births in 1918, the year of a serious influenza epidemic, then declined to 68 per 10,000 live births in 1921, and fluctuated between 65 and 70 per 10,000 live births throughout the 1920s.[40] Indeed, it was not until the mid-1930s that the maternal mortality rate began to show a significant decline. Nonwhite mortality rates remained twice as high as white rates during this period. Although exceedingly high between 1915 and 1933, infant mortality rates per 1,000 live births declined 40 percent, and neonatal mortality rates per 1,000 live births declined 10 percent. In contrast, maternal mortality rates during the same period never dropped below 61 per 10,000 live births.[41]

Professional and popular literature published after 1915 on the subject of maternity increasingly emphasized how shocking it was that so many women were dying at the time of their "greatest usefulness to the state and to their families," and how American ignorance, fatalism, and apathy concerning the perils of childbearing had made the United States one of the worst places in the world in which to have a baby.[42] In 1930, the United States placed last among twenty-five countries to which it was compared. In comparison with advances made in reducing deaths associated with certain diseases and with efforts made toward improving infant survival, no progress had been made since the turn of the century toward improving maternal survival.

These reports also indicated that certain of the problems contributing to high maternal death rates were viewed as distinctively American. These included the inadequate numbers of properly educated professionals in maternity care; their lack of skill in conducting labor; the excessively interventionist stance of physicians; the maldistribution of physicians, which favored urban areas; the inaccessibility for reasons of transportation of health care services to rural women; racial heterogeneity; and poverty. Emphasizing that infant survival was dependent on maternal survival of pregnancy and childbirth, these reports stated that the most serious threat to the integrity of the family and the survival of the American nation was excessive *maternal* mortality in childbearing.[43]

Such events as the passage of the Sheppard–Towner Act in 1921 financing prenatal education and supervision and the establishment of committees to study maternal mortality also reinforced the view that childbirth for women was potentially even more dangerous than military service for men.[44] While the Twilight Sleep debate had provided impressionistic evidence of the degree to which women suffered in childbirth, maternal mortality statistics provided incontrovertible proof that childbirth and war were equivalent in terms of the casualties, fatalities, and anguish they each caused.[45] Although they disagreed on the reasons why, Americans could no longer view maternity as being as natural as breathing or sleeping. Maternity was a "bodily crisis" that demanded expert supervision.[46]

Accordingly, the period between 1915 and the Second World War was characterized, in part, by Americans' ardent efforts to prevent women from succumbing to what they saw as one of nature's most beautiful and most deadly phenomena. United in their belief that no woman should have to "ransom" her life in order to give life,[47] physicians, nurses, society women, lay reformers, and sensation-seeking journalists joined together to prevent the death and destruction that they saw awaiting every pregnant woman.[48]

Indeed, the new watchword in maternity care was *prophylaxis*. In general terms, prophylaxis meant the prevention of complications in maternity through the complete medical and nursing supervision of the pregnant woman from conception through several weeks postdelivery. Professionals advised women of the benefits of seeking assistance early. Professional assistance was intended to promote health and was based on the premise that most problems in maternity were preventable.

While prophylaxis also included such physical appraisal and laboratory screening techniques as blood pressure monitoring, pelvic measurement, and urine and blood analyses, it was primarily nonphysical and nontechnological in means and ends. That is, the aim of prophylactic measures, collectively referred to as prenatal care and primarily offered by nurses in the home and community settings, was to bring the woman to a state of health by such means as education, counseling, and reassurance where she would require little or no artificial assistance at birth. Advocates of prenatal care showed a recognition of the role such nonmedical factors as environment, income, and education played in affecting pregnancy outcomes. Accordingly, the prenatal "propaganda"[49] that increasingly appeared in popular magazines, government pamphlets, and health care facilities had a fairly comprehensive focus.[50]

Yet prophylaxis also had a distinctively different meaning and direction that eventually prevailed. Although he was not the first to articulate or practice it, Joseph DeLee (1869–1938) was the most important and influential advocate of this kind of prophylaxis. While the Twilight Sleep debate, the public dissemination of mortality figures, and women's own experiences of suffering in childbirth all contributed to a negative view of it in the natural state, DeLee was arguably the person most responsible for convincing professionals and the general public that childbirth was a potential biological nightmare for modern women.

In a landmark article, "The Prophylactic Forceps Operation," published in 1920, DeLee recommended the routine use of forceps, episiotomy, and the early removal of the placenta to protect the perineum and the baby's head from injury and to conserve the woman's energy.[51] It was clear to DeLee that most of the damage done in labor was caused by the trauma of the fetal head pounding against the perineum and ultimately tearing it in the *natural* state. Asserting that "everything, of course, depends on what we define as normal," DeLee argued that if a woman were to fall on a pitchfork and rupture her perineum, that would be considered abnormal. If a baby's head were to be caught in a door, that would be considered abnormal. Yet, when in the course of every natural labor, a baby had to struggle against tight pelvic floor muscles, injuring or sometimes even killing either himself or his mother or both, that was considered normal. For DeLee, it was obvious that labor was as "pathogenic" as the accidents he cited, and anything that was pathogenic was by definition also "pathologic or abnormal." Significantly, for DeLee, if an event could cause disease, it had to be viewed *as* a disease.

Moreover, DeLee believed that women ought to be as "anatomically perfect" after delivery as they were before it for their own sakes and their husbands'.[52] In fact, a woman's genitalia could be restored to their "virginal" state by surgically incising the perineum *before* it had a chance to tear naturally. An artificial cut was so much cleaner and more controlled than a jagged, natural tear. The operation he recommended would, in his opinion, relieve the anguish of labor by shortening it, promote less bleeding and infection, prevent irreparable damage to the mother and infant, and, most importantly, supplement and anticipate nature's own somewhat flawed efforts. For DeLee, it was nature that made labor the morbid affair that it was, leading to widespread invalidism among women. Obstetric prophylaxis reduced the need for gynecologic treatment. DeLee revealed his abhorrence of natural labor best when he stated that he often wondered "whether Nature did not deliberately intend women to be used up in the process of reproduction, in a manner analogous to that of the salmon, which dies after spawning."[53]

In much of his written work and in the interviews he gave, DeLee emphasized how inefficient the modern woman's reproductive apparatus and nervous economy were in dealing with childbirth.[54] Lamenting that such factors as modern living, the mixing of the races, disease, and women's own horror of childbirth had made it essential for physicians to intervene in childbirth with drugs and instruments, DeLee mused that it was probably better for the health of the infant if all deliveries were by cesarean section rather than allowing it to struggle through the torturous passages of its mother's beleaguered genital tract. Natural labor endangered infants, and it produced untold anguish in the husbands who were so often left with "ailing, unresponsive" wives.[55] Prophylactic obstetrics was, accordingly, vital to women, infants, and marital harmony.

DeLee warned that the prophylactic use of drugs and instruments was safer than nature only in the hands of trained specialists. While he acknowledged that he was painting a grotesque picture of childbirth, he insisted that he was merely stating the facts as they were and as "modern science" had shown them to be. Indeed, DeLee did see scores of women suffer from both incompetent obstetric care and poor general health.[56] Accordingly, his view that the wise obstetrician expected things to go wrong was somewhat justified.

DeLee's prophylaxis contrasted sharply with the prophylactic measures offered primarily by the nurse. First, DeLee's prophylaxis focused on the event of childbirth itself and emphasized the mechanisms of parturition. In contrast, prenatal care focused on the entire pregnancy and emphasized the general health and well-being of women, including such factors as diet and mental attitude. Second, DeLee's prophylaxis emphasized pharmacologic and technologic intervention in the intrapartal and immediate postpartal periods, while nurses emphasized educative and emotive means to prevent complications as soon as pregnancy was confirmed. Third, while prenatal care could be intrusive in the sense that it frequently involved the imposition of the nurse's values upon a patient, DeLee's prophylaxis was physically intrusive and subjected women to iatrogenic complications in childbirth. Fourth, while prenatal care could largely be offered by any trained caregiver, DeLee's prophylaxis required a physician's expertise.

DeLee's espousal of the prophylactic forceps operation refueled the debate among physicians about the consequences of meddlesome midwifery, but the philosophy underlying the operation—namely, that of *routinely* anticipating and improving on the natural process of birth with drugs and instruments—became the basis for the modern specialty of obstetrics, which had fully emerged by the end of the 1930s. Yet DeLee eventually regretted the role he had played in promoting the abuse of prophylactic obstetrics when it was shown to be a major cause of birth-related accidents.

The most influential medical study of maternal mortality, the New York Academy of Medicine's 1933 report on *Maternal Mortality in New York City: A Study of All Puerperal Deaths, 1930–1932*, revealed that pain-relieving drugs and accompanying operative intervention were major causes of death.[57] The report's findings, which were carried by many newspapers and magazines in the country, indicated that the use of anesthesia in labor and delivery had become a "problem of the most pressing importance, more so in the United States than in any other country."[58] Its authors estimated that the rate of operative intervention in the United States was as much as 15 percent greater than the optimum. Citing the "easy accessibility of anesthesia" as the factor most responsible for the "frequent use of instrumentation," the authors noted that of all deaths investigated, 69 percent had involved the use of anesthesia. Furthermore, they indicated that the early termination of labor by artificial means was "casually regarded," especially in large cities where hospital facilities made this practice easy. Most importantly, the report acknowledged that, on the whole, physicians and hospitals were more frequently implicated in maternal deaths than midwives and the home.[59]

Although many physicians accepted the findings of the report, others attempted to show that women were at least as responsible for their injuries and deaths in childbirth as physicians. Several lines of argument emerged.[60] First, medical writers defending current personnel and practice argued that they were often unfairly held accountable for deaths that should have been attributed to midwives. Specifically, physicians were forced to attend women who were already in a moribund state because of their insistence upon having midwives deliver their babies.

Second, some physicians depicted themselves as being unduly subject to shifts in public attitudes about childbearing. They blamed the lay press for raising women's expectations to the point where they demanded miracles from their doctors. Moreover, if women had the fortitude and patience their grandmothers had, they would not be so obsessed with avoiding hardships in childbirth at any cost. According to these physicians, it was women's "phobia" about childbirth pain and their relentless quest for absolute painlessness in labor that had caused the "furor operandi" so characteristic of obstetric practice after 1915. Furthermore, it was the "layman's false sense of values" that forced physicians to derive profit from using drugs and instruments. If the public, according to this argument, had properly compensated physicians all along for *not* using them, their tendency to intervene would never have asserted itself so strongly.[61]

Third, some physicians subtly blamed women for their reproductive patterns. One physician implied that women had themselves caused the shift in value that made the infant's life equal to the mother's and, therefore, worthy of *any* efforts to save it by having fewer babies; and another suggested that women were not cooperating with their doctors unless they had their first babies in their early twenties. A first pregnancy in an older woman often required intervention.[62]

Although controversial and a proven cause of suffering and death, prophylactic obstetrics was clearly appealing to many physicians and struck a responsive chord with them for several reasons. Until the 1940s, childbirth *was* a hazardous event, no matter what the major explanation was. Since a woman carrying a child to term was most likely to die during the intrapartal and early postpartal periods (if she was going to die at all), it was not unreasonable to focus attention on what could be done at that time to avoid injury and death. Many physicians fervently believed that the prophylactic use of drugs and instruments halted the further deterioration of the modern woman and, through her, of the race at large. In their view, the artificiality of civilized life required artificial means to offset its negative consequences. Moreover, they believed that in expert hands prophylactic obstetrics was neither destructive nor radical but rather restorative and conservative. Drugs and instruments restored women to health, conserved their mental, emotional, and physical energy, and left them more able and willing to bear more children.[63]

Yet physicians appeared to have other, less altruistic reasons for adopting an interventionist stance. Prophylactic obstetrics offset what many physicians viewed as the pure "drudgery" and boredom of labor. Moreover, it was more efficient and economical for a physician, already hard-pressed for time, to be able to control the duration of labor.[64] Indeed, two frequently cited criteria for the *ideal* method of pain relief were that it not be too time-consuming and that it be easy for most physicians to use.[65]

Physicians emphasized how easy labor could be, not only for women but also for themselves with pain-relieving drugs and instruments. Arthur Bill, the Cleveland obstetrician who strongly advocated prophylactic obstetrics, preferred easing all labors by making them shorter with such techniques as the application of forceps. While he acknowledged, for example, that a fetal head in the posterior position would rotate to the normal anterior one by itself in the majority of cases, he preferred not to wait so that women would not suffer so much pain. Yet he paradoxically advocated the use of techniques to shorten labor that were themselves painful, suggesting that pain relief was not the sole motivation for using them.[66]

Significantly, Bill's article illustrates that prophylactic obstetrics included the infliction of pain for the ostensible purpose of reducing the natural pain of labor. Pain-relieving drugs allowed the physician to execute procedures, such as the intensification of uterine contractions with oxytoxic drugs, the manual dilatation of the cervix, the artificial rupture of membranes, and the manual removal of the placenta, which were themselves often more painful than the labor itself, even when analgesics were used. Moreover, for some physicians, giving an oxytoxic drug, for example, was like giving a narcotic because both were intended to alleviate suffering.[67] Accordingly, any prophylactic technique could be justified on the grounds that it relieved pain. Furthermore, the common practice of using general anesthesia to postpone delivery until the physician's arrival clearly indicates that control, rather than pain relief per se, tended to inform the use of pain-relieving measures.[68]

The prophylactic use of drugs and instruments also clearly separated the physician, especially the obstetric specialist, from midwives and nurses. In the early decades of the twentieth century, medicine as a whole was engaged in upgrading its standards and status.[69] Obstetricians, in particular, were acutely aware of the image problem obstetrics had because of high maternity-related morbidity and mortality rates. They attributed much of it to the fact that so many nonphysician caregivers were still providing maternity services to women. In their view, obstetrics would continue to be the "Cinderella" specialty and the "step-child" of medicine, if midwives, nurses, and others continued to operate independently.[70] Spurred on by the pivotal Flexner Report of 1910 (which found that the medical profession was in general overcrowded and undermined by the lack of uniform and rigid standards for educa-

tion and practice),[71] and J. Whitridge Williams' 1912 recom-
mendations for achieving obstetric reform,[72] obstetricians
sought to limit the numbers of individuals who could attend
childbearing women or to control the practice of those who did,
including general practitioners and nurses.

Using the public forum, including women's clubs and the lay
press, obstetricians launched a successful campaign to sell their
technical expertise to Americans. "Cultivat[ing] a professional
mystique" that maximized the value of the kind of prophylaxis they were practicing and minimized the value of prenatal care, obstetricians reversed the unfavorable image of the
meddlesome male midwife and emerged as concerned human-
itarians whose sole interest was maternal and infant welfare.[73] By the 1940s, they had replaced midwives as chief birth
attendants to all women and had relocated childbirth from the
home to the hospital.[74]

The minutes of the Ohio Obstetrical Society in the early
1930s indicate that physicians' efforts in maternity care were
often self-serving. These minutes reveal a great concern with
what the public thought of obstetricians and with gaining and
maintaining control of maternity services.[75] They show, in
particular, that physicians were willing to allow that some
women would not receive prenatal education, which they admitted was important, if they could not control this service.
For example, physicians wanted women to obtain their per-
mission to take a prenatal course offered by nurses. According
to one physician, nothing was so important as the

intervention of a third factor, and a nonmedical factor at that, between the patient and his physician. The relationship of the physician to his patient must not be disturbed, therefore the doctor should
in each instance contact the Academy (where the course was being
offered) and register his case for the course and that no case should
be accepted which did not present the Academy card.[76]

Physicians' opposition to and eventual defeat of the
Sheppard–Towner Act also revealed their fear that the preventive maternity services offered to women in their homes and
the community by nurses and others with government sup-

port threatened the physicians' claims to leadership and domination in obstetric care.[77]

In the 1950s, Leon Festinger described a phenomenon called cognitive dissonance that refers to the psychological discomfort individuals experience when exposed to contradictory facts, opinions, or beliefs about a situation or event in which they are highly invested.[78] According to Festinger, individuals achieve consonance by choosing to alter their own beliefs and by accepting new facts, or by choosing the more difficult alternative of redefining those other facts and beliefs to bring them in alignment with their own.

Prophylactic obstetrics was a response to the reality of suffering and death in childbirth, but it was also clearly a response to physicians' growing need to define childbirth solely in terms of suffering and death. Physicians were clearly uncomfortable with the fact that medical intervention was a major cause of morbidity and mortality in childbirth. Physicians were clearly uncomfortable with the fact that nurses and midwives could provide effective prophylactic services to maternity patients. Physicians were clearly uncomfortable with what they perceived as the low status of obstetric medicine in comparison to practice fields such as surgery.

Faced with evidence that drugs and instruments were often implicated in childbirth injuries and deaths and with the effectiveness of nonphysician caregivers in maternity—but eager to establish obstetrics as a scientific and prestigious medical specialty—physicians chose to emphasize the hazards of natural birth and the similarity between childbirth and other medically treatable conditions. Yet, by redefining childbirth in almost exclusively medical terms, physicians chose the more difficult path to psychological consonance. Since the practice of prophylactic obstetrics ultimately rested on nothing more scientific than physicians' claims that it was indeed scientific, physicians themselves along with prophylactic obstetrics remained vulnerable to continuing criticism.

Notes

1. Clifford B. Lull and Robert A. Hingson, *Control of Pain in Childbirth: Anesthesia, Analgesia, Amnesia* (Philadelphia: J. B. Lippincott, 1944), p. 115; Francis B. Wakefield, "Painless Childbirth," *American Journal of Obstetrics* 77 (May 1918):793–96.

2. Arthur H. Bill, "The Newer Obstetrics," *American Journal of Obstetrics and Gynecology* 23 (February 1932):159.

3. Nicholson J. Eastman, "Whither American Obstetrics?" *New England Journal of Medicine*, 16 January 1941, p. 93.

4. Howard W. Haggard, *Devils, Drugs, and Doctors: The Story of the Science of Healing from Medicine-Man to Doctor* (New York: Harper and Brothers, 1929), p. 3; S. P. Oldham, "Sacral Anesthesia in Obstetrics," *American Journal of Surgery* 39 (April 1925):45; and Wakefield, "Painless Childbirth."

5. Cited in the foreword to John J. Bonica, *Principles and Practice of Obstetric Analgesia and Anesthesia* (Philadelphia: F. A. Davis, 1972).

6. Walter Channing, *A Treatise on Etherization in Childbirth* (Boston: William D. Ticknor, 1848).

7. The problems described here were more or less known to physicians as soon as they started using drugs for pain relief. While they lacked detailed knowledge of maternal and fetal physiology, they, nevertheless, recognized the problems we recognize today as inherent to drug use in labor.

8. Mary C. Blackwell, "The Nursing Care of Obstetric Patients Having Anesthesia and Analgesia," *American Journal of Nursing* 33 (May 1933):425; Asa B. Davis, "Obstetric Analgesia," *Bulletin of the Lying-In Hospital of the City of New York* 13 (August 1928):231; and Thomas G. Gready and H. Close Hesseltine, "Continuous Caudal Anesthesia in Obstetrics: Preliminary Report," *Journal of the American Medical Association*, 23 January 1943, p. 230.

9. The gradual addition of more required routines in the care of the laboring woman is reflected in both medical and nursing literature. See, for example, successive editions of Joseph B. DeLee, *Obstetrics for Nurses* (Philadelphia: W. B. Saunders); Joseph B. DeLee, *The Principles and Practice of Obstetrics* (Philadelphia: W. B. Saunders); Carolyn Conant Van Blarcom, *Obstetrical Nursing* (New York: Macmillan); J. Whitridge Williams, *Obstetrics: A Textbook For the Use of Students and Practitioners* (New York: D. Appleton); and Louise Zabriskie, *Nurses' Handbook of Obstetrics* (Philadelphia: J. B. Lippincott). For the specific editions most used in this study and for changes in authors of these books, see the Bibliographical Essay. On the importance of these texts in the history of obstetric medicine and

nursing, see Eunice Claire Messler, "Transforming Information Into Nursing Knowledge: A Study of Maternity Nursing Practice" (Ed. D. dissertation, Teachers College, Columbia University, 1974), pp. 115–48; Harold Speert, *Obstetrics and Gynecology in America: A History* (Chicago: American College of Obstetricians and Gynecologists, 1980), pp. 128–29.

10. John J. Byrne, *A History of the Boston City Hospital, 1905–1964* (Boston: Sheldon Press, 1964), p. 222; Joseph B. DeLee, *The Principles and Practice of Obstetrics*, 2nd ed. (Philadelphia: W. B. Saunders, 1915), p. 300.

11. Lila J. Napier, "Nursing Care," *Trained Nurse and Hospital Review* 88 (May 1932):588; Bertha Van Hoosen, *Scopolamine-Morphine Anesthesia* (Chicago: House of Manz, 1915), see the photos between pp. 80–81 and 88–89; and Catherine Yeo, "Analgesia in Obstetrics II. Technic of Administration and Nursing Care," *American Journal of Nursing* 35 (May 1935):442.

12. Joseph B. DeLee, *Obstetrics for Nurses*, 5th ed. (Philadelphia: W. B. Saunders, 1918), p. 130.

13. D. N. Danforth, "Contemporary Titans: Joseph Bolivar DeLee and John Whitridge Williams," *American Journal of Obstetrics and Gynecology* 1 (November 1974):577–88.

14. DeLee, *Principles*, 1915, p. 300.

15. DeLee, *Principles*, 1920, pp. 303–8.

16. DeLee, *Principles*, 1925, pp. 312–18.

17. DeLee, *Principles*, 1929, pp. 312–18.

18. J. Whitridge Williams, *Obstetrics: A Textbook For the Use of Students and Practitioners*, 4th–6th eds. (New York: D. Appleton, 1917, 1925, and 1930), pp. 343–49, 359–65, and 386–94, respectively.

19. Arthur Bill, "The Choice of Methods for Making Labor Easy," *American Journal of Obstetrics and Gynecology* 3 (January 1922):65.

20. Arthur Bill, "Analgesia and Anesthesia and Their Bearing Upon the Problem of Shortened Labor," *American Journal of Obstetrics and Gynecology* 34 (November 1937):868.

21. H. W. Kostmayer, "A Practical Method of Minimizing the Pain of Labor," *New Orleans Medical and Surgical Journal* 69 (July 1916):89.

22. R. L. Raiford, "Painless Labor," *Virginia Medicial Monthly* 51 (June 1923):152.

23. C. O. McCormick, "Rectal Ether Analgesia in Obstetrics," *American Journal of Nursing* 33 (May 1933):415.

24. See the discussion following Raiford's article, "Painless Labor," p. 154.

25. William Gillespie, "Analgesics and Anesthetics in Labor: Their

Indications and Contra-Indications," *Ohio State Medical Journal* 11 (October 1915):612.

26. Philips J. Carter, "Pantopon-Scopolamine Seminarcosis in Labor," *American Journal of Obstetrics and Gynecology* 10 (November 1925):697.

27. Alan Frank Guttmacher, *Into This Universe: The Story of Human Birth* (New York: Viking Press, 1937), p. 207.

28. Herman L. Gardner, Harry Levine, and Meyer Bodansky, "Concentration of Paraldehyde in the Blood Following Its Administration During Labor," *American Journal of Obstetrics and Gynecology* 40 (September 1940):435–39.

29. Nicholson J. Eastman, "Apnea Neonatorum," *American Journal of Obstetrics and Gynecology* 40 (October 1940):647–51.

30. Edith L. Potter and Fred L. Adair, *Fetal and Neonatal Death* (Chicago: University of Chicago Press, 1940), p. 149.

31. Ibid.

32. James A. Harrar, "Rectal Ether Analgesia in Labor: Technic and Results in 5,800 Cases at the New York Lying-In Hospital," *Bulletin of the Lying-In Hospital of the City of New York* 13 (July 1927):159–66.

33. Blackwell, "Nursing Care of Obstetric Patients," p. 426.

34. Leonard Averett, "Nembutal and Scopolamine Analgesia in Labor, With a Report of 160 Cases," *American Journal of Obstetrics and Gynecology* 27 (January 1934):109–12; Waldo B. Edwards and Robert A. Hingson, "The Present Status of Continuous Caudal Analgesia in Obstetrics," *Bulletin of the New York Academy of Medicine* 19 (July 1943):516.

35. Howard F. Kane and George B. Roth, "The Use of Paraldehyde in Obtaining Obstetric Analgesia and Amnesia," *American Journal of Obstetrics and Gynecology* 29 (March 1935):366–69.

36. Austin Flint, "Responsibility of the Medical Profession in Further Reducing Maternal Mortality," *American Journal of Obstetrics and Gynecology* 9 (June 1925):865.

37. Oldham, "Sacral Anesthesia," p. 42.

38. Speert, *Obstetrics and Gynecology in America*, p. 146.

39. George Clark Mosher, "Maternal Morbidity and Mortality in the United States," *American Journal of Obstetrics and Gynecology* 7 (March 1924):294.

40. Monroe Lerner and Odin W. Anderson, *Health Progress in the United States, 1900–1960* (Chicago: University of Chicago Press, 1963), p. 32.

41. U.S. Department of Health and Human Services, National Center for Health Statistics, *Vital Statistics of the United States, 1977,*

Vol. 1. Natality (Washington, D.C.: Government Printing Office, 1981).

42. Grace L. Meigs, *Maternal Mortality From All Conditions Connected With Childbirth in the United States and Certain Other Countries*, U.S. Children's Bureau, Pub. 19 (Washington, D.C.: Government Printing Office, 1917), p. 9.

43. Beulah Amidon, "Women and Children Last," *Survey*, February 1938, pp. 38–39; S. Josephine Baker, "Maternal Mortality in the United States," *Journal of the American Medical Association*, 10 December 1927, pp. 2016–17; Mary Sumner Boyd, "Why Mothers Die," *Nation*, 18 March 1931, pp. 293–95; Dorothy Dunbar Bromley, "What Risk Motherhood?" *Harper's*, June 1929, pp. 11–12; Mary A. Clarke, "Maternal Mortality: Its Implications for the Nursing Profession," *Trained Nurse and Hospital Review* 92 (February 1934):151–56, 184; Susan M. Coffin et al., "Maternal Mortality in Massachusetts: A Study of 900 and 84 Deaths in the Puerperal State," *Journal of the American Medical Association*, 6 February 1926, pp. 408–13; Louis I. Dublin, "The Risks of Childbirth," *Forum* 87 (May 1932):280–84; "Maternal Care," *American Journal of Nursing* 31 (May 1931):599–600; Helena Huntington Smith, "Death at Birth: Our High Maternal Mortality," *Outlook*, 13 November 1929, pp. 405–8; U.S. Department of Labor, *Maternal Mortality in Fifteen States*, Children's Bureau, Pub. 223 (Washington, D.C.: Government Printing Office, 1934); and White House Conference on Child Health and Protection, *Obstetric Education* (New York: Century, 1932).

44. Sheila M. Rothman, *Woman's Proper Place: A History of Changing Ideals and Practices, 1870 to the Present* (New York: Basic Books, 1978), pp. 136–42; Jose G. Marinal, Alan L. Scriggins, and Rudolf F. Vollman, "History of the Maternal Mortality Study Committees in the United States," *Obstetrics and Gynecology* 34 (July 1969):123–38.

45. The analogy between childbirth and the battlefield, war, or military service continued to be commonplace at this time. See, for example, Paul De Kruif, "Why Should Mothers Die?" *Ladies Home Journal*, March 1936, p. 8.

46. "When Mothers Die It's News," *Nation*, 31 January 1934, p. 118.

47. J. C. Furnas, "That Mothers May Live," *Ladies Home Journal*, November 1939, p. 21. The author called the death of women in childbirth "murder for ransom" and equated their deaths to gassing thousands of people at once in Madison Square Garden.

48. Furnas and De Kruif are good examples of sensation-seeking journalists. See also Alice Kuehn, "Federation of Women's Clubs Undertakes General Campaign to Reduce Maternal Fatality," *Cleveland Plain Dealer*, 6 December 1936, Women's Magazine, p. 6; Katharine

F. Lenroot, "Safety for Mother," *Parents Magazine*, May 1935, p. 15; and A. J. Skeel, "Making Childbirth Safe in Cleveland," *Cleveland Clubwoman*, January 1937, pp. 6, 10–11 and February 1937, pp. 6, 10.

49. Furnas, "That Mothers May Live," p. 55.

50. For the educative and supportive focus of prenatal care and the nurse's role in offering it, see, for example, Shirley Hope Alperin, "The Maternity Center Association," *Nursing World* 134 (March 1960):14–16, 34; Frank W. Lynch, "A Child Is To Be Born," *Hygeia*, May 1926, pp. 253–55; and Anne Stevens, "The Public Health and the Extension of Maternity Nursing," *Public Health Nursing* 12 (June 1920):497–501. See also Maternity Center Association of New York, *Forty-Fifth Annual Report and Log, 1915–1963* (New York: Maternity Center Association, 1963), and pp. 60–71 of this book.

51. Joseph B. DeLee, "The Prophylactic Forceps Operation," *Transactions of the American Gynecological Society* (Philadelphia: William J. Dornan, 1920), pp. 66–71.

52. Ibid., p. 72; Joseph B. DeLee, "Obstetrics Versus Midwifery," *Journal of the American Medical Association*, 4 August 1934, pp. 309–10.

53. DeLee, "Prophylactic Forceps," p. 72.

54. Paul De Kruif, "Why Should Mothers Die?" *Ladies Home Journal*, March 1936, pp. 8–9, 101–8; April 1936, pp. 14–15, 108–9, 111, 114; May 1936, pp. 26–27, 91–92, 94, 96–97; and June 1936, pp. 28, 96–97, 99–100, 102; DeLee, *Principles*.

55. DeLee, "Obstetrics," p. 310.

56. Herbert Ratner, "The History of the Dehumanization of American Obstetrical Practice," in *21st Century Obstetrics Now!*, vol. 1, ed. Lee Stewart and David Stewart (Marble Hill, Mo.: N.A.P.S.A.C., 1977), pp. 115–46.

57. New York Academy of Medicine, Committee on Public Health Relations, *Maternal Mortality in New York City: A Study of All Puerperal Deaths, 1930–1932* (New York: Commonwealth Fund, 1933), pp. 113–27.

58. *The Commonweal*, 8 December 1933, pp. 143–44; "Causes of Maternal Mortality," *Literary Digest*, 12 February 1933, pp. 18, 116; "Hazards of Childbirth," *Nation*, 29 November 1933, p. 612; and "Why Mothers Die," *Time*, 27 November 1933, pp. 22, 24. According to "When Mothers Die It's News," *Nation*, 31 January 1934, p. 118, over three hundred newspapers in thirty-nine states picked up the story of the report.

59. New York Academy of Medicine, *Maternal Mortality*, pp. 113–27.

60. On the report and physicians' responses to it, see, for example, Joyce Antler and Daniel M. Fox, "The Movement Toward A Safe Maternity: Physician Accountability in New York City, 1915–1940," in *Sickness and Health in America: Readings in the History of Medicine and Public Health*, ed. Judith Walzer Leavitt and Ronald Numbers (Madison: University of Wisconsin Press, 1978), pp. 375–92. In general, physicians argued that U.S. statistics on maternal mortality were not so bad as they appeared because of the differences in computing these kinds of figures and because the United States had a greater racial mix bringing the rates up. See also Richard A. Balt, "Maternal Mortality Study for Cleveland, Ohio," *American Journal of Obstetrics and Gynecology* 27 (February 1934):309–13; Edward S. Brackett, "Observations on the Problem of Maternal Mortality," *New England Journal of Medicine*, 19 April 1934, pp. 845–51; and A. J. Skeel, "Obstetrical Society," *Bulletin of the National Association of Nurse Anesthetists* 6 (August 1938):110–16.

61. Roy P. Finney, *The Story of Motherhood* (New York: Liveright, 1937), pp. 3, 6–7; Guttmacher, *Into This Universe*, pp. 121, 225–27, 338; and J. McF. Bergland, "Changes in Obstetrical Procedure During the Last Thirty-Five Years," *Southern Medical Journal* 32 (February 1939):190.

62. Guttmacher, *Into This Universe*, p. 226; Aldine R. Bird, "Progress of Obstetric Knowledge in America: In Which Medicine Answers A Challenge," *Hygeia*, May 1933, pp. 437–38.

63. Bill, "Newer Obstetrics," pp. 155–64; Lull and Hingson, *Control of Pain*, pp. 112–13.

64. Joseph B. DeLee, "What Are the Special Needs of the Modern Maternity?" *Modern Hospital* 28 (March 1927):59–69; Brooke M. Anspach, "The Drudgery of Obstetrics and Its Effect Upon the Practice of the Art, With Some Suggestions for Relief," *American Journal of Obstetrics and Gynecology* 2 (September 1921):245; Kostmayer, "Practical Method," p. 91; and Raiford, "Painless Labor," pp. 152, 154.

65. Alfred M. Hellman, "The Alleviation of Pain During Labor," *American Journal of Nursing* 16 (September 1916):1197.

66. Bill, "Choice of Methods," pp. 65–71.

67. Max Davis, "Progress in Obstetrics," *American Journal of Nursing* 31 (July 1931):799–802.

68. F. A. Ditter, "Local Anesthesia in Obstetrics," *Northwest Medicine* 35 (April 1936):151. Ditter remarked that it was "doubtless" the experience of his colleagues to arrive at a multipara's delivery after the attendant had given her general anesthesia to prevent a precipitate delivery.

69. E. Richard Brown, *Rockefeller Medicine Men: Medicine and*

Capitalism in America (Berkeley: University of California Press, 1979); James G. Burrow, *Organized Medicine in the Progressive Era: The Move Toward Monopoly* (Baltimore: Johns Hopkins University Press, 1977); D. Kirschner, " 'Publicity Properly Applied': The Selling of Expertise in America, 1900–1929," *American Studies* 19 (Spring 1978):65–78; Gerald Markovitz and David Rosner, "Doctors in Crisis: A Study of the Use of Medical Education Reform to Establish Modern Professional Elitism in Medicine," *American Quarterly* 25 (March 1973):83–107; and Rosemary Stevens, *American Medicine and the Public Interest* (New Haven: Yale University Press, 1971).

70. A common metaphor for obstetrics was the "Cinderella" or "stepchild" specialty because of its low prestige. See, for example, Dublin, "Risks of Childbirth," p. 284.

71. Abraham Flexner, *Medical Education in the United States and Canada: A Report to the Carnegie Foundation for the Advancement of Teaching* (New York: Carnegie Foundation, 1910), pp. 117–18, for information on obstetrics.

72. J. Whitridge Williams, "Medical Education and the Midwife Problem in the United States," *Journal of the American Medicial Association*, 6 January 1912, pp. 1–7.

73. Burrow, *Organized Medicine*, p. 154.

74. Neal Devitt, "The Statistical Case for Elimination of the Midwife: Fact Versus Prejudice, 1890–1935 Part 1 and 2," *Women and Health* 4 (Spring and Summer 1979):81–96 and 169–86; Neal Devitt, "The Transition From Home to Hospital Birth in the United States, 1930–1960," *Birth and the Family Journal* 4 (Summer 1977):47–58; Judy Barrett Litoff, *American Midwives: 1860 to the Present* (Westport, Conn.: Greenwood Press, 1978); and Richard W. Wertz and Dorothy C. Wertz, *Lying-In: A History of Childbirth in America* (New York: Free Press, 1977).

75. Minutes of the Ohio Obstetrical Society, 1932–1937, Archives, Cleveland Health Sciences Library, Historical Division, Cleveland, Ohio.

76. Minutes, February 18, 1935.

77. Rothman, *Woman's Proper Place*, pp. 142–53.

78. Leon Festinger, *A Theory of Cognitive Dissonance* (Stanford, Calif.: Stanford University Press, 1957).

INTERLUDE: FROM PAIN
TO PLEASURE _____

After World War II, Americans directed their attention away from women's mere survival toward their satisfaction in childbirth. Probably the most important reason for this shift was the dramatic reduction in maternal mortality that had occurred. The greatest improvement in maternal survival took place between 1937 and 1945, during which the average rate of decline in mortality was unprecedented (and has not been duplicated since).[1]

Maternity care was no longer viewed as a "battle against invalidism and death."[2] Despite the continued existence of a significant mortality differential between white and nonwhite women, favoring the former, and of a variety of reports indicating that too many women still died from preventable maternity-related causes, by 1945 a general feeling prevailed that the battle had been won.[3] Maternity no longer represented a major threat to the health of American women. Physicians, in particular, claimed that the two major reasons for this were their assumption of the leadership role in obstetric care and the virtual elimination of home births.[4]

Yet along with the prevailing sense that childbearing was reasonably safe for women was the growing sense that it was not as satisfying for them or for their professional caregivers as it should be. Childbearing women, nurses, and physicians were concerned with how the new obstetrics had altered birth-giving. Americans' recent experiences with depression and war made the "regimentation" associated with hospital maternity care appear "unreasonable," inhumane, and even threatening to the security, emotional sustenance, and traditional values they hoped to rediscover in family life. As Hazel Corbin, a leading figure in nursing, argued, the family was the foundation of America's strength, and maternity, in turn, was the foundation of the family. Accordingly, maternity care had to be changed to accommodate a society in dire need of nurturance.[5] Significantly, childbearing women, nurses, and physicians indicated that the victory against suffering and death in childbirth may have been won at the expense of both personal and professional fulfillment.

The Advent of Psychosomatic Medicine

In the 1930s, psychiatrists and other physicians began to voice their concern that medical practice had become too narrowly focused on germs, body organs, and spectacular treatments instead of on the personhood of the patient. These physicians sought to recapture the *whole* patient and to preserve the intimacy of a physician-patient relationship eroded by the increasing medical reliance on technology and other health care professionals.[6]

In 1935, Flanders Dunbar published a ground-breaking survey of the literature on mind-body interactions. Concluding that "organicistic thinking" had led physicians to detach organs from the rest of the body and, in effect, to forget the person who housed them, she emphasized the role of psychic factors in the etiology of disease.[7] Dunbar was instrumental in inaugurating what was perceived as a "new era" in medicine—one characterized by serious efforts to eliminate the arbitrary and false dichotomy that had evolved between mind and body and between organ and organism.[8] Recognizing that much discomfort and disease did not respond to conventional organ-directed therapy, and also alarmed at the large numbers of apparently healthy men who were rejected or discharged from military service during World War II for psychiatric reasons, many physicians welcomed the "new" *psychosomatic* approach to the prevention, diagnosis, and treatment of illness. Indeed, they suggested that Americans' newly found leisure time, improved physical health, and rising expectations had contributed to more "pains," "ailing," and "unhappiness" than ever before—a paradoxical state that the psychosomatic approach both acknowledged and attempted to treat.[9]

The psychosomatic approach was not really new but rather very similar to the one that Hippocratic physicians had used and that modern physicians had gradually discarded.[10] Advocates of the psychosomatic approach called it the "old art" of healing in the new "machine age" of medicine; a "conceptual" approach that reemphasized the wholeness, integrity, and fluidity of the human organism; and "as old as Plato and as modern as the atom bomb."[11] Like Plato, physicians lamented the "great error" they had made in treating human beings by separating the "soul from the body."[12] Adherents of the psychosomatic approach exhibited a new respect for the pre—twentieth-century physician who knew considerably less about specific organ pathology and treatment than his modern counterpart but knew considerably more about his patient. They also revealed their new appreciation of the multiple causation of disease and espoused the "ecological principle in medicine" according to which human beings could not be properly viewed apart from their personal histories and environment.[13]

If the psychosomatic approach was not entirely new, the theoretical basis for it was. What was novel about the approach was the attempt to substitute a "scientific basis for things sensed intuitively by the physician."[14] By the mid–1940s, physicians had a much better understanding of the physiological effects of the mind and the psychological effects of the body. Advances in neuroanatomy, neurophysiology, and endocrinology, as well as the renewed interest in the work of such pioneering investigators as Walter Cannon and Ivan Pavlov, provided physicians with more convincing evidence of the mind-body link they had always assumed existed.[15]

Not only did the further demonstration of the neuroendocrine connection between *psyche* and *soma* clarify how an emotion such as fear could cause organic changes in the body, but it also provided the biologically oriented psychology of

Sigmund Freud with a stronger scientific basis. Indeed, a key characteristic of the physicians who described and advocated the psychosomatic approach in medical practice throughout the 1940s and 1950s was their psychoanalytic orientation.[16]

While physicians who cared for childbearing women and women with reproductive disorders had always commented on the close connection between a woman's mental and emotional status and her unique body functions, modern obstetrician-gynecologists initially resisted the psychosomatic method when it was introduced in the 1930s. At the height of their campaign to make obstetrics, in particular, as respectable and scientific a medical field as surgery, these physicians were apparently reluctant to incorporate such an unmeasurable and subjective a factor as emotion into their practice. Several physicians noted the lack of cooperation and sympathy between obstetricians and psychiatrists.[17]

Yet, by the 1950s, obstetrician-gynecologists demonstrated a keener interest in the psychosomatic approach. William S. Kroger, a "dynamically oriented gynecologist," and S. Charles Freed, an endocrinologist, both with little training in psychiatry, published in 1951 the first important text surveying psychosomatic gynecology and obstetric literature.[18] They indicated that although their colleagues had become interested in the method later than physicians in other fields of medicine, they were, nevertheless, in the best position to practice it because so many of their patients' problems were "based on psychosexual disorders." Moreover, they stated that most gynecologists readily acknowledged that a large percentage of their patients were "neurotic" or had "nothing wrong with them" organically, even if they did not necessarily act on this knowledge.[19] Other medical literature also revealed a growing rapprochement between obstetrics and psychiatry.[20]

The work of such key psychoanalysts as Therese Benedek helped to shift obstetricians' attentions to the minds of their patients, but it was primarily the work of Helene Deutsch that provided physicians with a theoretical basis for their rather long-standing belief that the center of a woman's mental and emotional life lay in her reproductive organs.[21] In fact, few works on the psychology of women were cited more frequently in both professional and lay literature throughout the 1940s and 1950s than Deutsch's two-volume book on the subject published in 1944 and 1945.[22] According to Deutsch, menstruation, maternity, and menopause were among the most interesting "psychosomatic problems" there were. During a conference on the psychological aspects of childbearing, Deutsch declared that the female endocrine system was a "grandiose machinery of 'compliance' for the various psychic contents [and] emotional conflicts."[23] Most importantly, for Deutsch, there was no clear line between normality and deviance in the matter of women's psychology since the normal woman was herself perceived as operating on the basis of character traits that too frequently became exaggerated: masochism, narcissism, and passivity.

By the early 1950s, many physicians saw no clear distinction between the practice of obstetrics-gynecology and psychiatry. For them, the physician who treated women for their reproductive problems was also treating their minds since so much of the symptomatology encountered in these patients was of "purely mental origin."[24] While they lamented the overly pathological perspective of childbearing that had made the experience a surgical event, they still demonstrated a distinctively pathological perspective of their own. More precisely, they still viewed childbirth as a condition that required expert medical supervision. One physician said it best when he labeled pregnancy as "primarily an emotional problem."[25]

Maternity emerged as a maturational crisis of the highest order, demanding constant mental surveillance and prophylactic intervention. Even in the psychosomatic context, (and because of the continuing problem of postpartum psychosis), the childbearing woman was not really normal but rather "apparently normal" or "so-called normal."[26] According to Gerald Caplan, a leading figure in mental health, the "anticipatory guidance" of the pregnant woman was like an "emotional vaccination" against the threat of mental illness.[27] More importantly, since physicians saw the childbearing woman as the key biological and psychic link between generations, they assumed that preventing mental illness in her was the best way to prevent it in society as a whole.[28]

The advent of psychosomatic medicine in the 1930s reflected a medical awareness that something important was
missing in the practice of medicine that ultimately hurt both
patients and physicians. Those physicians who advocated the
incorporation of the psychosomatic approach into medical care
were concerned with how much the science of medicine had
interfered with the practice of its art. While obstetricians, in
particular, used the method to varying degrees, they were also
concerned with what has come to be known as the "medicali-
zation" of the childbearing experience. At the very least, many
of them acknowledged the importance of psychological variables to medically safe and emotionally satisfying obstetric
outcomes.[29]

Yet the psychosomatic method had a paradoxical effect on
obstetric care. On the one hand, its emphasis on the importance of maternity as an emotional (not merely physiological)
experience for women directed physicians to see childbirth in
a somewhat less disease-oriented way. Its emphasis on the
importance of psychological evaluation and treatment of the
childbearing woman directed physicians away from an exclusive focus on physical or technological diagnostic and treatment measures. Talking to a pregnant woman and allowing
her to express her feelings could be just as effective in preventing labor complications as forceps or episiotomy.

On the other hand, the psychosomatic approach merely
reinforced the view that childbearing was not a wholly normal
state. It was still a condition, albeit an emotional one, that required medical surveillance and treatment. In short, the psychosomatic approach humanized the relationship between
physician and childbearing woman, but it did not move childbearing out of the medical realm.

The Dilemmas of the Obstetric Nurse

Standing somewhat unobtrusively between the childbearing
woman and her physician was the obstetric nurse who ultimately shouldered the greater burden of implementing both
prophylactic obstetrics and the psychosomatic method.[30] From
her emergence as a separate type of nurse in the late nine-

teenth century through the 1950s, the obstetric nurse was the physician's "lieutenant"—on the front lines of the battle against illness, death, pain, fear, and boredom in childbirth.[31]

The obstetric nurse primarily protected the childbearing woman from the hazards of misinformation, anxiety, and loneliness through prenatal supervision, education, and support offered in the home and by community agencies. Also importantly, the obstetric nurse protected her patient from infection, hemorrhage, and other complications by her painstaking attention to aseptic technique and her constant surveillance during the confinement and lying-in periods. And the obstetric nurse was the caregiver who protected the patient from the dangers of anesthesia and analgesia in labor by providing a safe environment. In short, it was primarily the nurse who comforted, counseled, and cared for the childbearing woman, providing her with the most constant professional attention of any caregiver in the maternity cycle.[32]

Prior to the incorporation of pain-relieving drugs as a routine part of obstetric care, what the nurse did for the patient by preparing her body and mind for childbirth defined the limits of relief. As physician Edward Davis noted in 1917, since there was "little or nothing which the physician can do for his patient" in the first stage of labor, it fell "under the care of the nurse."[33] Moreover, the nurse protected the patient from the potential excesses of physicians. Suggesting that the physician's presence in the first stage encouraged women to demand drugs that only delayed labor and suffering further, Davis stated that it was better for the physician to be absent until delivery.

When the use of pain-relieving drugs in labor became routine, nurses administered these drugs and then supervised the patient afterward. While the use of these drugs had initially extended the physician's involvement in childbirth beyond the delivery period to include the first stage of labor, physicians increasingly delegated the tasks associated with their use to nurses. Medical and nursing literature directed at nurses gradually included more detailed information on the uses, side effects, and methods of administration of pain-relieving drugs and the care of the patient under their influence. By 1941, a

contraindication to offering pharmacologic pain relief to laboring women was having *no* nurse available to care for them.[34]

The obstetric nurse emerged with the founding of maternity
hospitals, the establishment of separate departments of obstetrics in general hospitals, and the growing recognition of the
importance of good maternity care for the public health and
welfare.[35] She was a distinctively American product intended
to perform virtually all of the duties of her European counterpart—the trained midwife—without being called a midwife and
without in any way undermining physicians' aspirations toward attaining and keeping the leadership role in maternity
care. Responding to the "midwife" title like a "bull . . . to a
red rag,"[36] and viewing both trained and untrained midwives
as potentially threatening to the establishment of medical he-
gemony in the field of maternity care, physicians increasingly
turned to nurses who were already being educated to "supplement," "support," and "augment" but not to "duplicate" the
services of the physician.[37] Trained to assist him in his presence, to substitute for him in his absence, but never even to
attempt to replace him, the nurse appeared to the physician
as the best solution to the problem of how to provide obstetric
care to all of the women who needed it, especially those who
were out of the easy reach of or unattractive to physicians.[38]

In fact, the trained nurse was viewed as the physician's
"missionary" in the urban tenements and rural hovels of the
nation, "spreading the gospel of good obstetrics" on his behalf.[39] Groomed to be subservient to the physician, nurses were
successfully courted by physicians as the ideal persons to bridge
the gaps, fill the breach, and step into the voids made even
wider by medical efforts to limit the numbers of professional
practitioners in obstetrics, to transfer childbirth from the home
to the hospital, and to pursue well-paying clientele. Even when
they were assisting women to give birth miles away from a
physician, nurses were expected to think of themselves as mere
extensions of the physician's eyes and hands and as performing their duties under his direction.[40]

Physicians extolled the virtues of the trained nurse as the
best answer to the "midwife evil."[41] Like the midwife, the
trained nurse let nature take its course. Like the midwife, the

trained nurse acted as a sister and warm companion to the childbearing woman. And like the midwife, the trained nurse was especially suitable to assist women who were ignorant and poor. Moreover, the trained nurse relieved the physician of the most "irksome parts" of obstetric practice, saved him time, and was a profitable addition to obstetrics for the physician.[42]

Accordingly, physicians argued that by replacing the midwife with the trained obstetric nurse, the *physician* could offer *all* women scientific obstetric care as well as the "sisterly service" the midwife used to provide without an appreciably greater expenditure on the physician's part of effort or money. In fact, since the nurse was obliged to act for him whenever he was unavailable, the *physician* could provide scientific and sisterly care without being with the patient at all.

Physicians courted nurses, but they were also clearly afraid of the nurses' potential for dislodging physicians from their preeminent place in maternity care. Physicians sought to reassure each other that nurses did not aspire to practice obstetrics independently. Believing that nurses did not want the responsibilities of interpreting symptoms and initiating treatments, but then knowing that it was nurses' responsibility to recognize normality and deviance in childbirth and to begin treatment when complications occurred, physicians demonstrated their reluctance to acknowledge the *de facto* independence of nurses on whom they increasingly relied to practice obstetrics. In 1904, one physician stated that it was the nurse's "delight" not to operate independently of the physician, and another physician in 1959 stated that nurses would be "most unhappy as . . . independent practitioner[s] of midiwifery."[43]

Physicians' need for nurses but fear of them placed nurses in a precarious position with physicians. Assigned duties that did not *belong* to them, but for which they were, nevertheless, responsible whenever physicians wanted them to be, nurses often found themselves forced to choose between their allegiance to their patient and the patient's physician. In addition to their nursing duties, nurses were obliged to see that physicians performed their duties properly, to help physicians appear in a favorable light to the public, and to make the practice of obstetrics easier for them.[44]

For example, according to one set of directives, the duties of the nurse were greatly increased in cases where physicians were not overly careful in adhering to aseptic technique.[45] Having painstakingly and scrupulously cleansed, shaved, gowned, and draped the patient and having cleansed, gowned, gloved, and groomed herself, the nurse was forced to resort to "tact" and to "example and precept" when working with a physician who was lax about asepsis.[46]

According to another directive, the physician was to be notified as soon as possible if labor occurred in the daytime and early evening hours, but he was not to be called until labor was active during the night.[47] Physicians frequently indicated that they did not want to be called until the "head is about ready for delivery," but medical writers also warned nurses never to permit a "precipitate" delivery, defined as one that occurred in the physician's absence. Nurses were sometimes instructed to perform the dangerous act of preventing the expulsion of the fetus by such techniques as keeping the patient's legs together or keeping a hand over the vulva to delay birth until the physician arrived.[48] To be sure, competent medical practitioners frowned upon these practices. Yet physicians were, for the most part, also eager to be present at and in control of what most people viewed as the climactic moment in the maternity cycle—perhaps to justify their presence in the labor room at all. Unwilling simply to wait for the moment to arrive, physicians made the topic of "when to summon the doctor" one of the most crucial elements in the proper training of the obstetric nurse.

The obstetric nurse was also a key factor that allowed the transfer of childbirth from the home to the hospital and eased the entry of obstetrics into a "newer operative era."[49] Recognizing the value of having everything they needed to learn and to practice obstetrics in one location, physicians depended on nurses for a variety of technical and managerial services. If advances in antisepsis, anesthesia, and surgical techniques made the nurse important in the home, they made her vital in the hospital that advertised skilled nursing services and scientific care as its advantages.[50] Moreover, the nurse was obliged to make the hospital more acceptable to the maternity patient. She was the woman's hostess away from home, providing her with "womanly sympathy" and making her forget she was not at home.[51]

The good obstetric nurse had to be properly educated. Yet a constant dilemma for physicians was exactly how much education was good for her and, more importantly, for physicians. Again, physicians acknowledged the need for nurses to be *at least as proficient as physicians* since so much of obstetric care was delegated to them. Yet physicians feared the influence that education offered nurses. Physicians shared knowledge with nurses but warned them never to think of themselves as better than physicians. Moreover, many leading physicians were clearly incensed by nurses' aspirations to control their own education and by the development of nursing examinations that asked questions *even doctors* could not answer.[52]

From most indications, physicians really had nothing to fear from nurses who accepted the demanding but obsequious role that physicians and prevailing cultural norms concerning the proper role of women in health care expected them to play.[53] Clearly recognizing and proud of the value of their services to maternity patients and to the advancement of obstetric medicine, nurses typically reassured physicians that they did not intend to supersede them in the care of the childbearing woman, nor did they intend to encroach upon medical territory or embarrass the physician in any way. Eager to establish themselves as valuable professionals, nurses warned each other not to miss the opportunity of becoming the physician's first and best assistant. Nurses even expressed their willingness to forgo attempts to meet patient needs if that meant threatening physicians in any way.[54]

The good obstetric nurse never felt safe about a mother or baby until she had transferred both into the physician's hands. The good obstetric nurse knew that it was more important for her to prevent an "untimely" delivery than to attempt it herself. The good obstetric nurse was the one who "calls most loudly for a doctor." The good obstetric nurse knew "her limitations." Most importantly, the good obstetric nurse knew her worth but did not flaunt it.[55]

The few nurses who expressed themselves directly on the

subject viewed the use of pain-relieving drugs in labor as a boon to the childbearing woman but as a somewhat mixed blessing for themselves. Agreeing with the prevailing view of childbirth as a period of severe pain during which women faced the possibility of injury and death, some nurses saw the introduction of these drugs into obstetric care as humane and in harmony with their goal of minimizing the discomfort of the laboring woman. Some identified with the infant and viewed the pain of childbirth as more than compensated for by the child's birth. Other nurses identified with maternity patients as women and viewed the pain of childbirth as less than tolerable when agents existed that could relieve it. For hospital nurses, in particular, the patient was "fortunate" to receive anesthesia and "happy" to deliver her child without remembering much about her ordeal.[56]

Yet nurses also expressed some ambivalence about these drugs. On the one hand, drugs were perceived as making the care of the laboring patient qualitatively better, easier, and more interesting. Moreover, some nurses suggested that the use of these drugs enhanced the value of the nurse to the patient and physician—both of whom depended on nurses for their safe use. Several brief reports from medical journals in the *American Journal of Nursing* of 1914 and 1915 highlighted the importance of the nurse in the care of the Twilight Sleep patient and the special training she required to assist physicians with the treatment.[57] In a sense, they suggested that the nurse with special skills was herself special. Other nurses remarked how much more manageable the labor patient under the influence of drugs was. Such a woman was quieter and disturbed other patients much less. More importantly, these nurses suggested that there was a "satisfying element" in being able to *do* something to comfort their patients, implying that nurses had some difficulty dealing with labor patients' distress.[58]

By the 1930s, nurses also noted that the responsibility for providing pain relief was a difficult one for them. Mary Blackwell remarked how hard it had become for the nurse to determine labor progress in the patient under the influence of drugs and, thus, difficult to determine when to summon the doctor.

Warning nurses to sharpen their observational skills when caring for these patients, Blackwell revealed that often the nurse's desire to make certain that she was not calling the physician unnecessarily was "accompanied by a precipitate delivery."[59]

Instructional literature for nurses also indicated that the administration of certain pain-relieving regimens was much more difficult than some physicians claimed. For example, contrary to physicians who asserted that the administration of rectal analgesia was easy enough for "even" the student nurse to perform, descriptions of the method show that it required considerable effort on the part of the laboring woman and skill on the part of the nurse.[60] Prior to the development of an apparatus that allowed the installation of medication into the bowel against gravity within a few seconds, the procedure could last up to thirty minutes. The laboring woman was required to lie on her side and to overcome her natural urge to expel the fluid, and the nurse was obliged to control the installation in such a way that fluid only passed into the bowel between contractions. The nurse was also obliged to perform the entire procedure with a minimum of soiling to prevent contamination of the genitals, which predisposed women to puerperal infection.[61]

Also clear from nursing literature is the fact that contrary to some physicians' claims that patients were not overly excited when they received amnesic drugs in labor, nurses were forced to resort to restraints. A notable feature in instructional literature for nurses on obstetric anesthesia and analgesia, written by nurses, is their increasing emphasis on the nurse's role in protecting the patient from harming herself and the consequences for the patient if she did not.[62]

Nurses were also obliged to appeal to women for their cooperation prior to receiving drugs. While nurses could not give their opinion one way or the other concerning the use of these drugs in labor, nurses were supposed to gain the patient's confidence, since a confident and calm patient allowed the drugs to work more effectively.[63]

A subtle but ultimately very damaging aspect of drug use for the nurse was her high visibility in relation to the procedures, which became necessary as a result of drug use. The nurse was the one who placed the patient in restraints or in a padded bed. The nurse was the one who separated a woman from her family and stripped her of her personal belongings, specifically, hairpins, dental bridges, and jewelry that could harm her while under the influence of drugs. The nurse was the one who cleansed her, shaved her, purged her, prevented her from eating or drinking, and, in general, performed those carefully circumscribed routines demanded by the practice of prophylactic obstetrics. In fact, the nurse was the most visible agent of the strange, frightening, and often painful routines imposed on the laboring woman, if only because the nurse spent the most time with her. Most importantly, nurses now inflicted pain at least as often as they relieved laboring women of it. As both childbearing women and nurses moved from the home to the hospital for childbirth and to practice obstetric nursing, nurses began to appear less like sisterly companions in labor and more like unfeeling robots.

If women viewed physicians as indifferent to their suffering in childbirth, they viewed nurses as direct causes of it. Popular literature carried women's reports of the cruelty, callousness, and brutality of nurses.[64] One former hospital maternity patient saw the nurse as having the greatest "control" over patients, suggesting that women saw nurses, not physicians, as being responsible for the negative features of hospital care.[65]

Throughout the 1940s and 1950s, nurse writers increasingly acknowledged the extent to which they were failing to provide maternity patients with the care they really needed and wanted. Nurses admitted how indifferent they were to women's pain and how "mechanical and machine-like" they had become in their attitude to care.[66] Hazel Corbin, a long-term director of the Maternity Center Association of New York, remarked that nurses, like physicians, were providing care to "cases," instead of to whole people, to the "body," instead of to the "whole personality."[67] A major nursing figure in shaping an organization that had emphasized the humanistic aspects of maternity care since 1918, Corbin recognized that professionals had reached a point of diminishing returns by emphasizing the pathology rather than the normality of childbearing. Moreover, Corbin suggested that nurses had been thwarted by physicians in their attempts to provide nursing care. According to her, there was something very wrong when nurses, the largest group of health care providers, were unable to control their own activities. Warning nurses that unless they worked for "radical" change, they would remain nothing more than the physician's eyes and hands, Corbin challenged nurses to defy the status quo in obstetric care.[68]

Other nurses also indicated their growing understanding of what they had lost by following a mechanistic and pathological orientation. Nurses, even more than physicians, attempted to incorporate the psychosomatic approach into their care with patients.[69]

The dilemmas of the obstetric nurse should be viewed against a background of changes in American nursing as a whole. The most significant change was what David Wagner has called the "proletarianization of nursing"—a gradual process that hurt nursing more than benefited it.[70] Up until the 1930s, the trained nurse was primarily a private entrepreneur who enjoyed a fairly intimate relationship with her patient. Although the closeness of the relationship and the nurse's location in the patient's home were factors that presented unique problems of their own, nurses had considerable professional autonomy even though under the legal and nominal supervision of physicians.[71] Moreover, for a major portion of the period from the emergence of the trained nurse in the nineteenth century to the 1930s, what the nurse offered the patient in terms of physical care, emotional sustenance, and environmental control defined the limits of both care and cure. As one historian put it, the nurse was the one who had something to offer the patient.[72]

The discovery of specific causes of disease and effective remedies to treat them, such as antibiotics for infection, and the development and refinement of technological and surgical innovations in medicine shifted the balance of value to the physician and to the hospital—the science-based and technologically equipped workshop over which he presided. What the physician had to offer the patient now *appeared* more important and more scientific than what the nurse offered. More-

over, the depression made it economically untenable for nurses
to continue to do free-lance work, and the advent of third-party
payment to cover hospital costs forced hospitals to find a skilled
but manageable staff to care for their growing patient population.

While it is impossible to include all of the details of the
change here, by the mid–1940s, the majority of nurses had
become wage laborers in hospitals. Historians still debate the
consequences of the move from the home to the hospital and
the shift in emphasis from care to cure for nurses, but they do
agree that nurses lost most of the independence and self-
control they once had. Moreover, by uncritically accepting more
and more tasks delegated to them by physicians, without the
decision-making power to determine whether those tasks should
be carried out at all, nurses became more firmly entrenched
within the medical sphere than ever before.[73]

In the case of maternity care, in particular, nurses moved
from "center stage" to being upstaged by physicians in the
hospital. A 1963 study of the interrelationships among professional groups and patients revealed the lower-status positions
nurses *and* childbearing women gradually occupied vis-à-vis
physicians who directed the events of childbearing and then
starred at delivery itself.[74]

This upstaging of both nurses and childbearing women suggests a distinctive dilemma that the obstetric nurse increasingly faced apart from those she shared with other nurses.
Recent scholarship has focused on the dilemma that derives
from the problematical relationships women have with each
other in a male-defined world, which values the masculine and
devalues the feminine. Judith Bardwick described the "alter-
nating cycle of intimacy and repudiation" that characterizes
women's relationships.[75] Sara Lightfoot depicted mothers and
school teachers as reluctantly engaged in the "alien" task of
perpetuating sexist norms in the home and classroom.[76] And
Mary Daly, writing about female caregivers and women patients, described nurses as "token torturers" of women on physicians' behalf.[77] In short, these scholars and others view women
as "common victims of sexism"[78] or as suffering from a minor-

ity group self-image which leads them to dislike and suspect each other.[79]

The common-victims approach is a useful one for understanding the evolving relationship between nurses and childbearing women. It emphasizes how devalued groups struggle against each other instead of with each other against the sources of their devaluation. It explains why nurses, eager to gain professional prestige, accepted the tasks of prophylactic obstetrics and the values that informed it so easily. It suggests why nurses, even more than physicians, were viewed as cruel and brutal and as initiators of many prophylactic routines. One woman said it best when she told her readers in a 1937 book on prenatal advice to remember that if they were "lonely" as patients in hospitals, nurses were "more lonely."[80]

The Displeasures of the Childbearing Woman

The impetus for changing maternity care seems to have come primarily from childbearing women themselves. Professional literature indicated that it was the "consumer" who was "rebelling" against the way in which obstetrics was being practiced and demanding more personalized treatment.[81]

Yet the transfer of childbearing from the home to the hospital occurred with women's consent. To be sure, physicians had waged a successful campaign in the 1920s and 1930s outlining the dangers of nonphysician-directed home deliveries. In addition, such factors as the virtual elimination of midwives as birth attendants and the concentration of medical and nursing personnel in hospitals served to reduce women's choices in childbearing.

Many women, however, were attracted to the scientific care offered them in hospitals and were eager for the one-or two-week respite from the responsibilities of family life as well as the responsibility for preparing the home for confinement.[82] Middle- and upper-class women made the hospital the preferred place of childbirth in the early 1930s. By the end of the 1940s, the greater availability of and accessibility to maternity beds in hospitals, the prevailing assumption that hospital care was directly responsible for the dramatic improvement in maternal health, and the elimination of midwives made the hospital the preferred place of childbirth for all women. By 1950, 88 percent of all births were in hospitals.[83]

Moreover, women continued to want safe and effective pharmacologic pain relief, which required hospital care. Constance Todd's well-researched and polemical 1931 book on the Gwathmey method of obstetric analgesia was almost identical in its arguments to the literature published by Twilight Sleep advocates fifteen years before.[84] Proselytizing the advantages of pharmacologic oblivion in childbirth, women's right to demand it, and physicians' reluctance to give it to them, Todd's book appeared during the height of physicians' campaign to place childbirth firmly within the domain of medical practice. Continuing to emphasize women's suffering in childbirth and their consequent need for physicians to relieve it, writers such as Todd made the selling of prophylactic obstetrics—featuring physicians, hospitals, drugs, and instruments—that much easier. A 1933 *Parents Magazine* article also extolled the virtues of the Gwathmey method, and a 1937 book on prenatal advice extolled the virtues of hospital care and encouraged women to be sure to choose a physician who believed in obstetric anesthesia, suggesting that there continued to be physicians who were reluctant to use it.[85]

Moreover, through the 1940s and 1950s, women continued to express their gratitude at being able to sleep through childbirth. More importantly, there is very little evidence to suggest that women ever felt themselves to be *more* expert than their doctors in the matter of childbearing.[86]

Yet there were also women who expressed their disappointment with hospital maternity care and with drug-induced oblivion in childbirth, in particular; and it was their point of view that gained momentum in the 1950s. These women described the "scattering of consciousness" and the "complete shattering of individuality," states akin to "death," which they experienced with amnesic drugs.[87] More significantly, these women clarified the separation between the sensations arising from the physiological process of labor itself and the psychological and environmental context in which these sensations were felt.

One woman, in a 1939 *Atlantic Monthly* feature, described her "struggling for consciousness" while under the influence of drugs as worse than any pain.[88] Another woman, in a 1939 *American Mercury* article, argued against "painless childbirth," induced by drugs, and for "conscious childbirth," in which the pain women felt allowed them to experience "ecstasy" and "exaltation."[89] For these women, pain-relieving drugs in labor violated the "spirit and meaning of birth."[90] They preferred "clarity of sensation" to the "mere negation of physical unpleasantness."[91] Most importantly for these women, pain-relieving drugs in labor minimized the sensation of labor itself but paradoxically caused more suffering.

Popular literature in the 1940s and 1950s continued to show these themes and women's growing dissatisfaction not only with drugs but also with what they viewed as the brutal, nightmarish, and cruel experience of birth-giving in hospitals.[92] Women expressed disappointment with themselves, displeasure with their professional caregivers, and, most importantly, a rising expectation that what was supposed to be the greatest experience in a woman's life live up to its promise.

In the 1940s, the American woman became once again the subject of intensive scrutiny in both professional and popular literature. Perceiving her as the savior of American culture *and* its greatest threat, investigators of all kinds sought to establish her natural function, maternity, as the "cement" of American culture, one that would ultimately ensure an end to domestic conflict, the victory of democracy, and the rediscovery of "fundamental truths."[93]

Agnes Meyer, a mother of five and a grandmother of eight, asserted that the American woman, as mother, had the primary responsibility for stopping the moral decay in American society. "Democratic civilization" depended on the triumph of the truly feminine, that is, maternal woman. According to Meyer, the real and potential consequences of industrialization and communism made it vital that the modern woman "recapture . . . the wisdom" of assuming her main task and her "greatest honor," namely, the "vocation of motherhood." While a woman could successfully "sublimate" her "mother-instinct" in a career, she could only live "in the fullest sense" by conceiving, gestating, delivering, nursing, and rearing children of her own.[94]

The renewed emphasis on maternity as a woman's raison d'être and the "demographic debauch" that took place after the war, causing the American birth rate to rise to unprecedented levels, were apparently the results of a profoundly felt need to make up for the deprivations of war and the horror of the atomic bomb by extolling the richness and vitality of family life.[95] In addition, there was an economically motivated desire to control women's unprecedented invasion of the work place. Americans appeared determined to explain and thereby avoid those domestic problems that were weakening the American way of life against anti-American forces. The rediscovery of Freudian ideas about femininity, functionalist analyses of the family, and anti-Communist propaganda provided the rhetoric and ideology in the 1940s and 1950s, which made woman, as mother, the stable hub of an unstable universe. As procreators and guardians of the race, women were idealized as the most effective deterrents to crime and delinquency, family dissolution, mental illness, and war.[96]

If critics of American women exposed their failures as mothers or their failure to become mothers a sufficient number of times, it was only because it was logical to assume that if women were the primary deterrents to domestic and global conflicts, they were also the primary causes of them. Ferdinand Lundberg and Marynia Farnham, in their 1947 book *Modern Woman: The Lost Sex*, explained that women's health, prestige, and self-esteem derived from motherhood. To thwart the passive, inner-directed, and submissive characteristics of a woman's nature was to thwart nature itself. Women *had* to submit to their nature, epitomized in maternity, or they would continue to have the unhappy influence on society that had already produced such mass aberrations as communism, fascism, feminism, and the neurotic consumption of laxatives and cathartics.[97]

Historian Lynn White asserted that the American college woman had a special duty to ensure a stable population. The "creeping sterility" that was overtaking the more economically and intellectually endowed woman was a threat to democracy. According to White, the "unfulfilled task" of higher education for women was to instill in them the idea that it was both an "incentive" and a "duty" to bear at least three children in order to counteract the "drift toward totalitarianism."[98] Anthropologist and social biologist Ashley Montagu extolled the natural creativity of the womb and psychiatrist R. Coughlan found it a hopeful sign that modern women were becoming feminine again by having so many babies.[99]

Popular writers were also telling women that the journey from condemnation to praise could be accomplished by having babies. A 1956 *Life* feature chronicled the accomplishments of the American woman—the most "spectacular" of which was having babies.[100] Indeed, it was deemed so important for women's development and society's welfare that women have children, one woman indicated her willingness to undergo surgery if she had to prior to her marriage to ensure her fertility.[101]

In short, the woman living in the age of the "feminine mystique" from the 1940s to the early 1960s was perceived as instinctively moving toward only one goal in life—motherhood. According to Betty Friedan, who described this mystique, there was no other way for American women to "dream of creation or of the future" except to anticipate and repeat the experience of childbearing.[102] In view of the fact that many women who gave birth missed the experience of childbirth altogether, the rhetoric and ideology of maternity and the growing belief that the ordinary experiences of life ought to be savored to the fullest led these women to ask of their childbearing experiences, "Is that all there is?"

Notes

1. Monroe Lerner and Odin W. Anderson, *Health Progress in the United States, 1900–1960* (Chicago: University of Chicago Press, 1963), p. 33.

2. Louise E. Zabriskie, "Maternity Nursing in Hospital and Home," *American Journal of Nursing* 29 (October 1929):1157.

3. U.S. Department of Health, Education, and Welfare, National Center for Health Statistics, *Vital Statistics Rates in the United States, 1940–1960* (Washington, D.C.: 1968), p. 296. For a report on

maternal mortality, see, for example, Maternal Mortality Committee of the Committee on Maternal Health of the Minnesota State Medical Association, "Minnesota Mortality Study," *Minnesota Medicine* 27 (June 1944):475–81 and (July 1944):557–62.

4. See, for example, John H. Moore, "Maternal Mortality in North Dakota," *Journal of the American Medical Association*, 26 April 1941, pp. 1887–89. These claims are still disputed. See, for example, Neal Devitt, "Hospital Birth Versus Home Birth: The Scientific Facts, Past and Present," in *Compulsory Hospitalization: Freedom of Choice in Childbirth?*, vol. 2, ed. David Stewart and Lee Stewart (Marble Hill, Mo.: N.A.P.S.A.C., 1979), pp. 477–504.

5. Hazel Corbin, "Changing Maternity Services in a Changing World," *Public Health Nursing* 42 (August 1950):427–34.

6. Stanley Joel Reiser, *Medicine and the Reign of Technology* (Cambridge: Cambridge University Press, 1978).

7. Flanders Dunbar, *Emotions and Bodily Changes: A Survey of Literature on Psychosomatic Interrelations, 1910–1953*, 4th ed. (New York: Columbia University Press, 1954), p. 551.

8. Ibid., introduction from 1935 ed.

9. Francis J. Braceland, "Psychiatry—Psychosomatic Medicine and the General Practitioner," *Medical Clinics of North America* (Philadelphia: W. B. Saunders, 1950), pp. 939–55; William F. Hunter, "The Psychic Component of Pain in Gynecology and Obstetrics: A Sensory Conditioning Process," *American Journal of Obstetrics and Gynecology* 54 (November 1947):849, 853; *Kentucky Medical Journal* 43 (February 1945): 52; and Frank G. Slaughter, *Medicine For Moderns: The New Science of Psychosomatic Medicine* (New York: Julian Messner, 1947), p. 1.

10. The "humoral" theory of disease attempted to account for many phenomena in causation. See, for example, E. Ackerknecht, *A Short History of Medicine* (New York: Ronald Press, 1955), pp. 42–57.

11. Edward Weiss and O. Spurgeon English, *Psychosomatic Medicine: The Clinical Application of Psychopathology to General Medical Problems* (Philadelphia: W. B. Saunders, 1943), p. 1; Roy R. Grinker and Fred P. Robbins, *Psychosomatic Case Book* (New York: Blakiston, 1954), preface; and Slaughter, *Medicine for Moderns*, p. 1.

12. Stanley Cobb, *Borderlands of Psychiatry* (Cambridge: Harvard University Press, 1943), p. 3.

13. Smith Ely Jelliffe, "The Ecological Principle in Medicine," *Psychoanalytic Review* 35 (October 1948):367–88. This is a reprint of a 1937 publication by Jelliffe, considered to be the father of American psychosomatic medicine. He was a neurologist, then a psychoanalyst. See Karl A. Menninger and George Devereux, "Smith Ely Jel-

liffe—Father of Psychosomatic Medicine in America," *Psychoanalytic Review* 35 (October 1948):350–63.

14. Leonard G. Rowntree, foreword to *Psychosomatic Diagnosis*, by Flanders Dunbar (New York: Paul B. Hoeber, 1943), p. viii.

15. Cobb, *Borderlands of Psychiatry*, pp. 149–57.

16. Franz Alexander, *Psychosomatic Medicine: Its Principles and Applications* (New York: W. W. Norton, 1950); Felix Deutsch, ed., *The Psychosomatic Concept in Psychoanalysis* (New York: International Universities Press, 1953); and Weiss and English, *Psychosomatic Medicine*.

17. Louis Cohen, "Psychiatric Aspects of Childbearing," *Yale Journal of Biology and Medicine* 16 (October 1943):77; Karl A. Menninger, "Somatic Correlations With the Unconscious Repudiation of Femininity in Women," *Journal of Nervous and Mental Diseases* 89 (April 1939):523; and Howard C. Walser, "Fear, An Important Etiological Factor in Obstetric Problems," *American Journal of Obstetrics and Gynecology* 55 (May 1948):799.

18. William S. Kroger and S. Charles Freed, *Psychosomatic Gynecology: Including Problems of Obstetrical Care* (Philadelphia: W. B. Saunders, 1951), p. 3.

19. Ibid., pp. 1–2.

20. William C. Menninger, "The Emotional Factors in Pregnancy," *Bulletin of the Menninger Clinic* 7 (January 1943):15; Dwight M. Palmer, "Psychosomatic Orientations in Obstetrics and Gynecology," *Ohio State Medical Journal* 45 (October 1949):965.

21. Therese Benedek and Boris Rubenstein, *The Sexual Cycle in Women: The Relationship Between Ovarian Function and Psychodynamic Processes* (Washington, D.C.: National Research Council, 1942).

22. Helene Deutsch, *The Psychology of Women Volume I. Girlhood* and *The Psychology of Women Volume II. Motherhood* (1944; 1945; reprint ed., New York: Bantam Book, 1973).

23. Helene Deutsch, "An Introduction to the Discussion of the Psychological Problems of Pregnancy," in *Problems of Early Infancy*, ed. Milton J. E. Senn (New York: Josiah Macy, Jr., Foundation, 1948), p. 11.

24. Willard R. Cooke, "The Differential Psychology of the American Woman," *American Journal of Obstetrics and Gynecology* 49 (April 1945):457. See also William S. Kroger, "Psychosomatic Aspects of Obstetrics and Gynecology," *Obstetrics and Gynecology* 3 (May 1954):504–16.

25. Jere B. Faison, "Natural Childbirth," *Public Health Nursing* 43 (March 1951):121.

26. Fred D. Kartchner, "A Study of the Emotional Reactions During Labor," *American Journal of Obstetrics and Gynecology* 60 (July 1950):19; John Cooke Hirst and Flora Strousse, "The Origin of Emotional Factors in Normal Pregnant Women," *American Journal of the Medical Sciences* 196 (July 1938):98.

27. Gerald Caplan, "Psychological Aspects of Maternity Care," *American Journal of Public Health* 47 (January 1957):29.

28. Charles D. Kimball, "A Look Forward," *Bulletin of Maternal Welfare* 3 (March-April 1956):17–18; Samuel B. Kirkwood, "Complete Maternity Care," *American Journal of Public Health* 46 (December 1956):1547–52.

29. This will be developed in the discussion of Natural Childbirth in Chapters 4 and 5.

30. In this book, the obstetric nurse is the nurse who practiced obstetric nursing, although, in general, nurses did not practice along specialty lines exclusively. This is especially true for the private-duty nurse.

31. A. Worcester, "Obstetrical Nursing," *Boston Medical and Surgical Journal*, 17 January 1904, pp. 1, 4.

32. On the nurse's duties over the first half of the twentieth century see, for example, successive editions of Joseph B. DeLee, *Obstetrics For Nurses* (Philadelphia: W. B. Saunders); Carolyn Conant Van Blarcom, *Obstetrical Nursing* (New York: Macmillan); and Louise Zabriskie, *Nurses' Handbook of Obstetrics* (Philadelphia: J. B. Lippincott). See also Nell V. Belby, "Where and What Shall We Teach?" *American Journal of Nursing* 37 (January 1937):64–79; Committee on Education of the National League for Nursing Education, *Standard Curriculum for Schools of Nursing*, 1st, 4th, and 7th eds., rev. (New York: National League for Nursing Education, 1919, 1922, and 1927); Frederick H. Falls and Jane R. McLaughlin, *Obstetric and Gynecologic Nursing* (St. Louis: C. V. Mosby, 1937); Elizabeth Fishback, "Obstetrical Nursing as a Specialty," *American Journal of Nursing* 14 (July 1914):806–11; Helen F. Hansen, *A Review of Nursing: With Outlines of Subjects, Questions, and Answers*, 8th ed. (Philadelphia: W. B. Saunders, 1956), pp. 511–49; Mary E. Hutchison, "The Ward Patient at Sloane Hospital for Women, New York City," *Modern Hospital* 7 (September 1916):210–12; Jessie Lambert, "Obstetrical Work in the District," *Public Health Nurse Quarterly* 5 (April 1913):72–75; Henry F. Lewis, "Obstetrical Technique in the Cook County Hospital," *Surgery, Gynecology and Obstetrics* 2 (January 1906):81–82; Ruth E. Lindberg, "Clinical Instruction in Obstetrical Nursing," in *Clinical Instruction and Its Integration in the Curriculum*, 3rd ed., ed. Deborah MacLurg Jensen (St. Louis: C. V. Mosby, 1952), pp. 359–

409; Margaret McCulloch, "A Normal Home Delivery," *Trained Nurse and Hospital Review* 102 (May 1939):419–24; and Chelly Wassenberg and Ethel Northam, "Some Time Studies in Obstetrical Nursing," *American Journal of Nursing* 27 (July 1927):543–44.

33. Edward P. Davis, *Obstetric and Gynecologic Nursing*, 5th ed., rev. (Philadelphia: W. B. Saunders, 1917), p. 62.

34. Nicholson J. Eastman, "Remarks on Obstetric Anesthesia and Analgesia," in *Proceedings of the First American Congress on Obstetrics and Gynecology*, ed. Fred L. Adair (Evanston, Ill.: Mumm Print Shop, 1941), pp. 191–95.

35. Barbara Melosh, *"The Physician's Hand": Work Culture and Conflict in American Nursing* (Philadelphia: Temple University Press, 1982), pp. 113–57; Harold Speert, *Obstetrics and Gynecology in America: A History* (Chicago: American College of Obstetricians and Gynecologists, 1980), p. 15.

36. Hattie Hemsschemeyer, "Midwifery in the United States," *American Journal of Nursing* 39 (November 1939):1183.

37. Penelope K. Hope, "How the Public Health Nurse Assists the Obstetrician in the Care of His Patients," *Bulletin of Maternal Welfare* 3 (July-August 1956):16–18.

38. Hemsschemeyer, "Midwifery," pp. 1181–87; Maternity Center Association, *Twenty Years of Nurse-Midwifery, 1933–1953* (New York: Maternity Center Association, 1955); and Sister M. Theophane Shoemaker, *History of Nurse-Midwifery in the United States* (Washington, D.C.: Catholic University of America, 1947).

39. Joseph B. DeLee, *Obstetrics For Nurses*, 5th ed., rev. (Philadelphia: W. B. Saunders, 1918), p. 19.

40. Mary Breckinridge, *Wider Neighborhoods: A Story of the Frontier Nursing Service* (New York: Harper and Brothers, 1952); C. Lee Buxton, "Changing Attitudes in American Obstetrics," *Bulletin of Maternal Welfare* 5 (May-June 1958):7–11; Keith Folger, " 'A Quarter's Worth of Chloroform, Doctor,' " *Obstetrics and Gynecology* 4 (November 1954):588–90; Frederick W. Goodrich, "Modern Obstetrics and the Nurse," *American Journal of Nursing* 57 (May 1957):586–88; Ethel M. Tschida, "Can the Nurse Bridge the Gap Between the Hospital and the Home?" *Bulletin of Maternal Welfare* 5 (January-February 1958):23–25; and John Whitridge, "Nurse-Midwife Fills a Gap in Obstetric Care," *Modern Hospital* 93 (November 1959):95–98.

41. Iago Goldston, *Maternal Deaths—The Ways to Prevention* (New York: Commonwealth Fund, 1937), p. 41.

42. Buxton, "Changing Attitudes," p. 9; Gerald Caplan, "The Mental Hygiene Role of the Nurse in Maternal and Child Care," *Nursing Outlook* 2 (January 1954):14–19; Goodrich, "Modern Obstet-

rics," pp. 586–88; William T. McConnell, "The Trained Nurse in Obstetrics," *Southern Medical Journal* 16 (October 1923):792–99; George Gray Ward, "Our Obstetric and Gynecologic Responsibility," *Journal of the American Medical Association*, 3 July 1926, pp. 1–3; B. P. Watson, "Can Our Methods of Obstetric Practice Be Improved?" *Bulletin of the New York Academy of Medicine* 6 (October 1930):647–63; and Worcester, "Obstetrical Nursing," p. 2.

43. Worcester, "Obstetrical Nursing," p. 3; Whitridge, "Nurse-Midwife," p. 98.

44. Joseph Brown Cooke, *A Nurse's Handbook of Obstetrics*, 3rd ed., rev. (Philadelphia: J. B. Lippincott, 1907).

45. Herbert Marion Stowe, "The Specially Trained Obstetric Nurse—Her Advantages and Field," *American Journal of Nursing* 10 (May 1910):553.

46. Charles B. Reed, *Obstetrics For Nurses* (St. Louis: C. V. Mosby, 1923), p. 159; Stowe, "The Specially Trained Obstetric Nurse," p. 553.

47. J. Morris Slemons, "The Conduct of a Normal Labor at the Johns Hopkins Hospital," *Surgery, Gynecology and Obstetrics* 2 (February 1906):200.

48. DeLee, *Obstetrics for Nurses*, 5th ed., rev., p. 122; Reed, *Obstetrics for Nurses*, p. 147; and G. D. Shultz, "Journal Mothers Report on Cruelty in Maternity Wards," *Ladies Home Journal*, May 1958, pp. 44–45, 152–55. That nurses continued this practice through the 1950s is evident from the *Journal* report. Physician directives concerning when they wanted to be called and their definition of what a precipitate delivery was indicate that physicians viewed labor not solely in terms of its inherent physiology but rather in terms of their control over it. Moreover, as indicated in the previous chapter, anesthesia was used to delay delivery. See, for example, E. Seymour and Clifford E. Baldwin, "The Use of Spinal Anesthesia in Obstetrics at the Evanston Hospital," *American Journal of Obstetrics and Gynecology* 71 (May 1956):975. The authors stated that they did not use spinals to delay delivery, suggesting that other physicians continued to do so.

49. Stowe, "Specially Trained Obstetric Nurse," p. 554.

50. Jo Ann Ashley, *Hospitals, Paternalism, and the Role of the Nurse* (New York: Teachers College Press, 1976); Brian Little, "The Responsibility of the Teaching Hospitals to Practising Obstetricians," *Bulletin of Maternal Welfare* 3 (July-August 1956):23; E. D. Plass, "The Increase in Hospital Deliveries," *American Journal of Obstetrics and Gynecology* 40 (October 1940):659–61.

51. DeLee, *Obstetrics for Nurses*, 5th ed., rev., p. 444.

52. Cooke, *Nurse's Handbook*, p. 8; DeLee, *Obstetrics for Nurses*, 5th ed., rev., pp. 470–71; and George W. Kosmak, "Fundamental Training for Obstetric Nurses," *Transactions of the American Gynecological Society* (St. Louis: C. V. Mosby, 1927), pp. 72–84.

53. Ashley, *Hospitals*, pp. 75–93.

54. Louella Adkins, "The Care of an Obstetrical Patient," *American Journal of Nursing* 3 (June 1903):709–11; Mary E. M. Carter, "Maternity Care for the Moderately Well-To-Do," *American Journal of Nursing* 14 (February 1914):357–60; Katherine DeWitt, *Private Duty Nursing*, 2nd ed. (Philadelphia: J. B. Lippincott, 1917), p. 146; Carrie M. Hall, "Training the Obstetrical Nurse," *American Journal of Nursing* 27 (May 1927):373; and Isabel Hamptom Robb, *Nursing: Its Principles and Practice for Hospital and Private Use*, 7th ed. (Cleveland: E. C. Koeckert, 1916), p. 502.

55. Calvina MacDonald, "An Educational Program for the Nurse Which May Solve the Midwife Problem," Archives, 1927, University Hospitals of Cleveland, Cleveland, Ohio.

56. Mary C. Blackwell, "The Nursing Care of Obstetric Patients Having Anesthesia and Analgesia," *American Journal of Nursing* 33 (May 1933):427; Elizabeth Fishback, "Obstetrical Nursing as a Specialty," *American Journal of Nursing* 14 (July 1914):811; and Dorothy E. House, "The Patient in Labor," *American Journal of Nursing* 39 (December 1939):1333.

57. "Notes from the Medical Press," *American Journal of Nursing* 15 (February 1915):411 and "Twilight Sleep," *American Journal of Nursing* 14 (November 1914):88–89.

58. Anne Yelton and Marie Hilgediek, "Rectal Ether Analgesia from the Nurse's Standpoint," *American Journal of Nursing* 33 (May 1933):422.

59. Blackwell, "Nursing Care," pp. 425–27.

60. C. O. McCormick, "Rectal Ether Analgesia in Obstetrics," *American Journal of Nursing* 33 (May 1933):417.

61. C. O. McCormick, "A New Rectal Ether Analgesia Apparatus," *American Journal of Obstetrics and Gynecology* 20 (September 1930):411–13; James T. Gwathmey et al., "Painless Childbirth by Synergistic Methods," *Bulletin of the Lying-In Hospital of the City of New York* 13 (May 1924):83–94. This technique was in vogue in the 1920s and early 1930s.

62. Catherine Yeo, "Analgesia in Obstetrics II. Technic of Administration and Nursing Care," *American Journal of Nursing* 35 (May 1935):442; successive editions of Zabriskie's obstetric nursing text *Nurse's Handbook of Obstetrics*. In the 1952 edition, p. 320, there is

a photo of a patient with a chin bruise and a chipped tooth from having thrown herself against a radiator while under the influence of amnesics.

63. "Twilight Sleep," *American Journal of Nursing*, p. 88.

64. Shultz, "Journal Mothers Report," pp. 44–45, 152–55; Helen Washburn, *So You're Going to Have a Baby* (New York: Harcourt, Brace, 1937), pp. 61–62.

65. Ann Rivington, "Motherhood—Third Class," *American Mercury*, February 1934, pp. 160–65.

66. Ruth E. Owen, "Experiences in Childbirth—A Painful Ordeal," *American Journal of Nursing* 51 (January 1951):26.

67. Hazel Corbin, "A Nurse Looks Ahead," *American Journal of Obstetrics and Gynecology* 51 (June 1946):812.

68. This is from handwritten notes (probably Corbin's) in the Maternity Center Association of New York files in New York City. As part of an Institute on Maternity Nursing given in 1947, she spoke on "What is Maternity Nursing?"—the title on the cards.

69. Ellis J. Brandt, "Students Take A New Look—at the Obstetric Patient," *American Journal of Nursing* 56 (September 1956):1157–58; Hazel Corbin, "Maternity Nursing Education—Yesterday, Today, and Tomorrow," *Nursing Outlook* 7 (February 1959):82–84; Hazel Corbin, "Meeting the Needs of Mothers and Babies," *American Journal of Nursing* 57 (January 1957):54–56; Hazel Corbin, "Public Relations and Lay Support for Maternal and Child Health Goals," *Bulletin of Maternal Welfare* 5 (January-February 1958):7–11; Marion S. Lesser and Vera R. Keane, *Nurse-Patient Relationships in a Hospital Maternity Service* (St. Louis: C. V. Mosby, 1956); and Elizabeth Peck, "A Basic Collegiate Program in Maternity Nursing," *Bulletin of Maternal Welfare* 2 (July-August 1955):16–18.

70. David Wagner, "The Proletarianization of Nursing in the United States, 1932–1946," *International Journal of Health Services* 10 (1980):271–91.

71. Melosh, *Physician's Hand*, pp. 77–111.

72. Ashley, *Hospitals*, pp. 1–15.

73. Eva Gamarnikow, "Sexual Division of Labour: The Case of Nursing," in *Feminism and Materialism: Women and Modes of Production*, ed. Annette Kuhn and Ann Marie Wolpe (London: Routledge and Kegan Paul, 1978), pp. 96–123; Anselm Strauss, "The Structure and Ideology of American Nursing: An Interpretation," in *The Nursing Profession: Five Sociological Essays*, ed. Fred Davis (New York: Wiley, 1966), pp. 103–4.

74. William Rosengren and S. DeVault, "The Sociology of Time and Space in an Obstetrical Hospital," in *The Hospital in Modern So-*

Interlude: From Pain to Pleasure   83

ciety, ed. Elliott Friedson (New York: Free Press of Glencoe, 1963), pp. 266–92.

75. Judith M. Bardwick, *In Transition* (New York: Holt, Rinehart and Winston, 1979), pp. 133–52.

76. Sara L. Lightfoot, "Family-School Interactions: The Cultural Image of Mothers and Teachers," *Signs: Journal of Women in Culture and Society* 3 (Winter 1977):395–408.

77. Mary Daly, *Gyn/Ecology: The Metaethics of Radical Feminism* (Boston: Beacon Press, 1978), pp. 276–77.

78. D. Kravetz, "Women Social Workers and Clients: Common Victims of Sexism," in *Beyond Intellectual Sexism: A New Woman, A New Reality*, ed. Joan Roberts (New York: McKay, 1976).

79. Helen Mayer Hacker, "Women As a Minority Group," in *Female Psychology: The Emerging Self*, ed. Sue Cox (Chicago: Science Research Associates, 1976), pp. 156–70.

80. Washburn, *So You're Going to Have a Baby*, pp. 61–62.

81. Corbin, "Changing Maternity Servies," p. 428.

82. Richard W. Wertz and Dorothy C. Wertz, *Lying-In: A History of Childbirth in America* (New York: Free Press, 1977), pp. 154–64.

83. Louis Block, *Hospital Trends* (Chicago: Hospital Topics, 1956), p. 43; Neal Devitt, "The Transition From Home to Hospital Birth in the United States, 1930–1960," *Birth and the Family Journal* 4 (Summer 1977):47–58; and Donnell M. Pappenfort, *Journey to Labor: A Study of Births and Technology* (Chicago: University of Chicago Population Research and Training Center, 1964).

84. Constance L. Todd, *Easier Motherhood: A Discussion of the Abolition of Needless Pain* (New York: John Day, 1931).

85. Inis Weed Jones, "Childbirth With Less Pain and More Safety," *Parents Magazine*, February 1933, p. 19; Washburn, *So You're Going to Have a Baby*.

86. Constance J. Foster, "New Techniques in Childbirth," *Parents Magazine*, May 1940, pp. 24–25, 83–84; Marion Phillips, *More Than Pregnancy* (New York: Coward-McCann, 1955); and Joan Younger, *The Stork and You: A Guide for Expectant Mothers* (Philadelphia: Westminster Press, 1953).

87. M. Beatrice Blankenship, "The Enduring Miracle," *Atlantic Monthly*, October 1933, pp. 409–15.

88. Lenore Pelham Friedrich, "I Had a Baby," *Atlantic Monthly*, April 1939, p. 462.

89. " 'Painless' Childbirth I. A Mother Protests," *American Mercury*, June 1939, pp. 220–22.

90. "I Had a Baby Too," *Atlantic Monthly*, June 1939, p. 772.

91. Friedrich, "I Had a Baby," p. 462.

92. Shultz, "Journal Mothers Report." See also "From Genesis to Freud," *Nation*, 3 June 1936, p. 699 and "The Motherhood Bunk," *American Mercury*, November 1938, pp. 287–89.

93. Agnes Meyer, "Women Aren't Men," *Atlantic*, August 1950, pp. 32–33.

94. Ibid., pp. 32–36.

95. Landon Y. Jones, *Great Expectations: America and the Baby Boom Generation* (New York: Random House, Ballantine Books, 1981), p. 42.

96. Lois W. Banner, *Women in Modern America: A Brief History* (New York: Harcourt Brace Jovanovich, 1974), pp. 211–28; William Chafe, *The American Woman: Her Changing Social, Economic, and Political Roles, 1920–1970* (London: Oxford University Press, 1972), pp. 199–225; Peter Lewis, *The Fifties* (New York: J. B. Lippincott, 1978), pp. 42–64; Sheila Rothman, *Woman's Proper Place: A History of Changing Ideals and Practices, 1870 to the Present* (New York: Basic Books, 1978), pp. 224–31; and June Sochen, *Movers and Shakers: American Women Thinkers and Activists, 1900–1970* (New York: Quadrangle/New York Times Book, 1973), pp. 171–228.

97. Ferdinand Lundberg and Marynia Farnham, *Modern Woman: The Lost Sex* (New York: Harper and Brothers, 1947).

98. Lynn White, *Educating Our Daughters: A Challenge to the Colleges* (New York: Harper and Brothers, 1950), pp. 97–112.

99. R. Coughlan, "Changing Roles in Modern Marriaige," *Life*, 24 December 1956, pp. 108–18; Ashley Montagu, *The Natural Superiority of Women* (1952; reprint ed., New York: Collier Books, 1976).

100. "The First Baby," *Life*, 24 December 1956, pp. 57–63.

101. "Tell Me Doctor," *Ladies Home Journal*, April 1955.

102. Betty Friedan, *The Feminine Mystique* (1963; reprint ed., New York: Dell, 1970), p. 55.

THE QUEST FOR PLEASURE: THE NATURALIZATION OF CHILDBIRTH _____

In accord with the new psychosomatic approach, medical literature on the subject of pain in childbirth increasingly emphasized the *fear* of pain as the most important element of the pain experience. Professionals always recognized fear as integral to or associated with the pain phenomenon; but, in the mid–1940s, obstetrician-gynecologists (obstetricians) and other physicians and professionals began to view fear and its less defined partner, anxiety, as two of the most important clinical entities to be investigated, prevented, and treated in the childbearing woman. Indeed, she was seen as likely to have an almost overwhelming number of fears, notable among them, the fears of mutilation, of death, and of pain in childbirth.[1] The single most significant factor that both *generated* and *reinforced* American physicians' new interest in women's fear of childbirth and, in particular, their fear of pain in childbirth was the work of the British obstetrician, Grantly Dick-Read (1890–1959).

Read, who stated the theory, method, and goals of Natural Childbirth, believed that the modern woman had been subjected from childhood on to adverse mental conditioning concerning childbirth.[2] Mothers, women friends, husbands, the popular media, the Bible, history, and medicine itself had inadvertently conspired to create a profound fear of childbirth in women. This fear caused the muscular tension in labor that, in turn, made labor so painful. According to the theory of Natural Childbirth, the fear-tension-pain triad could be broken by eliminating the fear through individual and group educational and counseling sessions, and muscular tension could be reduced by teaching women certain psychophysical conditioning and relaxation techniques for use in pregnancy and labor. Read also believed the fear of childbirth could be prevented altogether by reeducating women, men, and children to view childbirth as a joyous and satisfying event—a natural experience that their distant female ancestors used to have without fear and, therefore, without pain. In short, the experience of Natural Childbirth involved the normal labor of an undrugged and fully informed woman. Although it was hard work, Natural Childbirth was not only a painless experience but also a pleasurable one for the woman who had no medical or obstetric complications interfering with the normal mechanism of birth, who was unafraid, mentally and physically prepared for childbirth, and surrounded by attendants who believed in the painlessness of a normal birth.[3]

Although Read's first American book, *Childbirth Without Fear: The Principles and Practice of Natural Childbirth*, was not published in the United States until 1944, there is some indication that a few Americans knew of his work as early as 1936. According to magazine writer Gretta Palmer, Blackwell Sawyer first used the Read method in 1943. Apparently called to the hospital bedside of a woman "screaming" in labor "at the moment" he was reading one of Read's books, this New Jersey "country doctor" quickly "applied" the Read method to the woman who, within one hour, delivered her baby with minimal pain and no anesthesia.[4] Pleased with this result, Sawyer continued to practice Natural Childbirth and subsequently wrote the first professional report on the actual use of the Read method in private practice to appear in an American medical journal. In the article, published in June of 1946, Sawyer described his favorable experiences with the method for 168 women he had delivered primarily in 1944.[5]

Furthermore, Read himself mentioned having received a letter from Joseph B. DeLee, then professor emeritus of obstetrics at the Universitiy of Chicago, in June of 1936, congratulating him on the publication of his first major work, *Natural Childbirth*, in 1933.[6] In the letter, DeLee promised to include Read's ideas in the next edition of *The Principles and Practice of Obstetrics*, which was published with the promised additions in 1938.[7] DeLee also mentioned having loaned Read's book to Paul De Kruif, the famous science writer, who, in turn, referred to Read's ideas in a very important series of articles on maternity in the *Ladies Home Journal*.[8]

Read also expressed his pleasure at having received a favorable review in the *Journal of the American Medical Association* of the *Revelation of Childbirth*, the British version of *Childbirth Without Fear*, published in 1942.[9] Moreover, the increasing incidence of articles in American professional and popular literature about the fear of childbirth and about the general mental and emotional status of the childbearing woman suggests that even if Read himself was not known in the United States before 1944, the ideas he espoused were.[10]

According to Read, very little attention had been given to the emotional factors in reproductive functioning anywhere prior to the 1933 publication of *Natural Childbirth*. Yet Read also acknowledged that he was "not really the originator of anything," that his theory and method of Natural Childbirth were not in the strict sense new.[11] In fact, virtually all of Read's major ideas had been more or less stated or implemented before. For example, as described previously, American physicians from the early nineteenth century through the early decades of the twentieth had stated their belief in the unnatural painfulness and natural painlessness of labor. While they may not have agreed with Read on the reasons why, physicians also believed that civilization had had a deleterious impact on labor. Moreover, like Read, few physicians failed to cite the real and potential dangers of providing pain relief in labor with drugs, failed to see the advantages of verbal suggestion in alleviating pain and its fear, or failed to see the connection between a woman's mental and physical state and the course of her labor.

Furthermore, the very existence of literature on prenatal advice prior to the advent of Read's method implies their authors' recognition of the value of preparation for childbirth. This literature included programs for the healthful management of pregnancy, and described the proper diet, exercise, clothing, and a variety of other preventive and remedial measures to ensure a safe and relatively painless delivery. Significantly, they also included advice on the maintenance of the proper mental attitude toward maternity.[12] Even those physicians who favored the routine use of pain-relieving drugs in labor re-marked that these drugs were more effective in women who were mentally prepared to receive them, relaxed, provided with appropriate physical and emotional support, and, most impor-tantly, unafraid.[13]

Finally, both advocates and critics of the Read method viewed it as a refurbished version of a way of giving birth that had passed. Read himself suggested that Natural Childbirth was the "psychosomatic" alternative to the "mechanistic" practice of obstetrics, and, as noted previously, the psychosomatic method was itself not really new.[14] The Maternity Center As-sociation of New York, a strong advocate of the Read method, indicated that when Read's book, *Childbirth Without Fear*, was first released in the United States, "it was apparent that his approach was similar to" the one the association had adopted since its beginning in 1918.[15]

While Read's theory and method of Natural Childbirth were in a number of ways familiar to Americans, there were also novel aspects. First, Read tied many previously stated ideas together in an organized fashion and provided a rational ex-planation of the assumptions on which they were based. Sec-ond, he included very specific breathing, exercise, and condi-tioning techniques, developed by the British physiotherapist Helen Heardman, with which women could use their own re-sources to combat fear and pain.[16] Third, and most distinc-tively, Read emphasized the pleasure of childbirth and the ex-perience of childbirth as a desired end in itself. For Read, childbirth was not merely an event a woman could have with a minimum of pain, but rather childbirth was a sublime and even spiritual experience. Contrasted with the prevailing American view that childbirth was an unfortunately neces-sary means to motherhood and one that required drugs to be tolerated at all, Read's ideas appeared not only novel but also heretical.

Accordingly, both the familiarity and the novelty of Read's ideas stimulated Americans' interest in them. On the one hand, Natural Childbirth was in harmony with the new psychosomatic trend in American medicine, and it evoked an image of a kind of childbirth experience that was somewhat nostalgic and romantic to Americans. On the other hand, Natural Childbirth also struck a discordant note with those who believed that the method was more metaphysical than scientific and that childbirth was an experience best controlled and best forgotten or wholly obliterated with drugs and instruments because of the suffering and damage it caused.

The Natural Childbirth Craze

Natural Childbirth became a significant milestone in American maternity care and a major American media event in a way that was very similar to the Twilight Sleep. Like the Twilight Sleep "furor," the Natural Childbirth "craze" was created by word of mouth, by the popular print media, by the demands of a growing number of women, and by the willingness of a growing number of physicians to satisfy them.[17] As suggested previously, relatively few Americans—except those who read one of Read's British books or papers, DeLee's 1938 textbook, or De Kruif's 1936 series in the *Ladies Home Journal*— knew of the Read method before Harper's published *Childbirth Without Fear* in 1944. It was not until 1948 that enough Americans knew of Natural Childbirth to make it an important part of American life. The Maternity Center Assocation of New York declared 1948 to be the year that "science join[ed] safety with serenity for safe and satisfying maternity."[18]

The beginning of the Natural Childbirth craze may be dated from when Blackwell Sawyer described his positive experiences with the method to Laurence Galton, a *Collier's* reporter, who popularized them for the general public in "Motherhood Without Misery," published in November of 1946. This article was, in turn, read by the pregnant wife of a medical student in New Haven, Connecticut, who subsequently arrived at the Grace-New Haven Community Hospital in labor and asked the assistant obstetric resident physician, Frederick W. Goodrich, if he knew of the Read method. He did, hav-

ing attended a medical meeting a month before at which it had
been discussed, and offered to assist her. The woman then delivered her baby successfully by Natural Childbirth. Her success, as well as that of over twenty women who asked for
"drugless delivery" at Grace-New Haven during the next few
months, apparently "sold" Goodrich and his superior, Herbert
Thoms, on the method.[19]

While Blackwell Sawyer has been referred to as a Read "pi-
oneer" and as Read's "foremost American disciple," it was
Herbert Thoms (1889–1972), the chief of the obstetric-
gynecology service at Yale University, who became the first
important American advocate, practitioner, and popularizer of
Read's method.[20] Indeed, it was Thoms who inaugurated the
first American Natural Childbirth program (the Yale program) in 1947 in cooperation with the Yale School of Medicine, School of Nursing, the Maternity Center Association of
New York, and his professional nurse and physician colleagues at Grace-New Haven.

Thoms met Read during Read's first tour of the United
States in 1947. Read, professionally ostracized and ridiculed
for his ideas in his native England, had been invited by the
Maternity Center in December of 1946 to speak at that association's annual meeting. On the evening of January 17, 1947,
Read presented his ideas before an audience of 2,500 people,
including nurses, physicians, other interested lay and professional people, and the press.[21] Thoms apparently met Read
during his New York engagement and then acted as Read's host
when he visited New Haven in February of 1947.[22] Thoms was
impressed by Read and his work and the successful use of
Read's method by a number of women who had delivered at
Grace-New Haven, but there were other factors that also led
him to advocate Natural Childbirth. Thoms was influenced by
the work of Helene Deutsch on the importance of psychological factors in the childbearing woman, and he was also located
in an institutional setting in which great strides had already
been made toward making the experience of birth more "family-centered" and toward the incorporation of the psychosomatic approach into maternity and pediatric care.[23]

Thoms started a pilot program in Natural Childbirth in 1947.

By the fall of 1948, he and Goodrich wrote the first report on the program for the *American Journal of Obstetrics and Gynecology*,[24] and virtually every major newspaper and popular magazine in the country carried the story of the successful Yale project and described the wonderful new way that women were having their babies in New Haven.[25]

Read's visits to other American cities were also well publicized by the popular press and by the Maternity Center and stimulated intense professional and public interest in his work. *Childbirth Without Fear*, which had not sold well at first, became a bestseller by the early 1950s,[26] and thousands of inquiries concerning Natural Childbirth poured into newspapers and magazines, Yale, and the Maternity Center.[27] One physician noted in 1950 how "one cannot go out to dinner without being asked about Natural Childbirth at Yale,"[28] and a journalist indicated in 1952 how difficult it was to handle the Natural Childbirth story "unsensationally."[29] After 1948, there was no doubt that Natural Childbirth had arrived in the United States.

Yet, while Natural Childbirth had become something of a household word, the term was being subjected to a growing number of different and even contradictory interpretations. Like the Twilight Sleep, Natural Childbirth always implied something more to Americans than a medical regimen designed to alleviate childbirth pain. Indeed, Natural Childbirth had many meanings. It was variously described in terms of the sensations or experiences of pain and pleasure, of the physical and psychological milieu in which birth took place, as a means to an end and as the end itself. Natural Childbirth was hailed as revolutionary, mildly praised as evolutionary, and vociferously condemned as retrogressive.

Accordingly, Natural Childbirth was equated with primitive childbirth, drug-free childbirth, painless childbirth, fearless childbirth, conscious childbirth, educated childbirth, and childbirth without artificial aid and with a normal result. Because such practices as breast feeding and rooming-in were closely associated with the method, Americans thought of them as being part of the method. The Maternity Center described Natural Childbirth as physiological birth achieved by a conscious woman with no artificial aid and no injury to mother or child.[30] A woman who described her experience of Natural Childbirth for the *Ladies Home Journal* stated that it was childbirth with pain and with ecstasy but without suffering.[31] A *Life* magazine article called it new *and* a "return to the natural age-old pattern of childbirth."[32] In contrast, two medical critics of the method called it old and the primitive and hazardous way women used to give birth before the advent of modern, scientific obstetrics.[33] Physician Nicholson Eastman and anthropologist Margaret Mead even suggested that Natural Childbirth was itself unnatural because it imposed "artifices," such as breathing routines, on the laboring woman.[34] In short, for Americans, there was no *single* theory, method, or set of goals in relation to Natural Childbirth.

Natural Childbirth versus Childbirth with Drugs

If Natural Childbirth meant anything at all to Americans after 1948, it was childbirth *without drugs* or with a *minimum of drugs*. In fact, the relatively drug-free aspect of Natural Childbirth was viewed as its most distinctive characteristic and as its greatest asset. Throughout the 1940s and 1950s, an even greater amount of space in professional journals and textbooks was allotted to the subject of obstetric analgesia and anesthesia. These editorials, literature reviews, and investigative reports on the use of pain-relieving drugs in labor included not only a greater variety of drugs and drug regimens but also an increasing number of directions, indications and contraindications, prohibitions, and warnings concerning their use. Physicians who authored this literature, for the most part, usually favored the use of pain-relieving drugs in childbirth and the availability of so many different drugs and drug regimens. However, they also commented on the striking lack of unanimity in the selection of techniques, and they recognized how complicated it had become for the physician to make the right choice to ensure safe and effective pain relief. Both professional and popular literature carried articles on the dangers of pain-relieving drugs in labor and highlighted the "price" women often paid for pain relief in labor.[35]

Most significantly, reports on maternal mortality that appeared in professional journals from the mid–1940s through the early 1960s indicated that obstetric anesthesia had become a leading cause of maternal deaths. In summary, these reports revealed that anesthesia deaths were almost always preventable and attributable to poor professional practices. Moreover, while the absolute numbers of maternal deaths due to obstetric anesthesia were relatively small, the decreasing incidence of deaths due to hemorrhage, infection, toxemia, and heart disease (the four major causes of maternal deaths) highlighted the extent to which anesthesia had emerged as a significant cause of women's deaths in childbirth. Even more importantly, anesthesia deaths frequently involved completely healthy women having normal births.

In addition, these reports indicated that the real incidence of maternal deaths due to obstetric anesthesia was obscured because they were usually not listed as anesthesia deaths in statistics collected on maternal mortality. Despite the critical fact that the "most common medical situation requiring anesthesia [was now] the delivery of a pregnant mother," the vast majority of hospitals did not have adequate anesthesia services, facilities, or equipment for maternity patients.[36] Furthermore, a medical career in obstetric anesthesia brought the physician little prestige and insufficient financial reward, thus attracting few qualified individuals, and physicians did not fully appreciate or use the services of trained nurse anesthetists or anesthesiologists. Finally, these reports demonstrated that while improvements had been made in obstetric anesthesia techniques, one anesthesia problem often replaced another as new techniques appeared and were widely used. For example, some reports noted that maternal deaths due to inhalation anesthesia were decreasing, but deaths caused by spinal anesthesia were increasing.[37]

Accordingly, those who advocated Natural Childbirth stressed how much safer the method was for women and their babies than childbirth. with pain-relieving drugs. Reports on the method showed that it was superior to childbirth with drugs on such medical criteria as length of labor (shorter in Natural Childbirth), incidence of spontaneous delivery (greater in Natural Childbirth), incidence of operative delivery, including cesarean sections and forceps manipulations (lower in Natural Childbirth), extent of maternal blood loss (decreased in Natural Childbirth), length of maternal convalescence (shorter in Natural Childbirth), and incidence of infant respiratory distress (lower in Natural Childbirth). In short, advocates of Natural Childbirth argued that the method was superior to childbirth with drugs on the usual medical measures of maternal and infant morbidity and mortality and obstetric outcomes.[38]

Natural Childbirth enthusiasts also emphasized how favorably the method ranked in comparison to childbirth with drugs on such psychological criteria as happiness, fulfillment, satisfaction, sense of esteem, and sense of achievement. They stressed the subjective value to women and their families of a method that allowed women to be active participants in the birth process, fully awake and conscious of every sensation of childbirth, and witnesses to their babies' births and first moments of life. According to advocates, Natural Childbirth strengthened the parent-infant and marital relationships, and it also provided the physicians and nurses who attended childbearing women with a more satisfying professional experience. In contrast to patients under the influence of drugs, Natural Childbirth patients were cooperative, willing and able to help themselves, and pleased and unafraid to give birth. Furthermore, advocates believed that pain-relieving drugs that obliterated women's memory or sensation of childbirth cheated them of the most important event of their lives—a consequence from which a woman might never recover. In short, Natural Childbirth advocates argued that the method was superior to childbirth controlled with drugs on the equally (if not more) important but difficult to measure criteria of pleasure.[39]

While the relatively drug-free aspect of Natural Childbirth was perceived as its greatest asset, in view of the actual and potential dangers associated with routine drug use in labor, it was also perceived as its greatest liability. Advocates of the method emphasized its drug-free safety, but critics warned of its drug-free dangers. Several themes emerged in the arguments of Natural Childbirth critics. First, they viewed Natural Childbirth as retrogressive. Natural Childbirth was accordingly, a rejection of both physicians and science and a denial of the progress made in maternal and infant care, which critics believed was, in part, directly attributable to physicians and the increased use of pain-relieving drugs. Some critics insisted on equating Natural Childbirth with the "natural" births women had who were unfortunate in having no one to help them or who received poor obstetric care. In addition, for some critics, when women asked for Natural Childbirth, they were also asking to suffer and die the way their grandmothers had.[40]

Second, Natural Childbirth was viewed as dangerous because it interfered with what was perceived as sound obstetric practice, meaning intervention with drugs and instruments. Physicians who advocated drug use in labor believed that pain-relieving drugs prevented the physician from intervening *prematurely* merely to satisfy the importunities of hysterical women and anxious family members to end the labor. For these physicians, drugs provided safe and comfortable labors for women and "controlled working conditions" for themselves.[41] In contrast, a 1949 *New York Times* article reported one physician's fear that Natural Childbirth would lead to an increase in maternal and infant morbidity and mortality because it discouraged physicians from assisting women who used the method. This physician implied that Natural Childbirth caused the physician to intervene *too late*.[42]

Third, Natural Childbirth was viewed as dangerous to the emotional health of women. Some described the "disillusioned Cinderella[s]"[43] the method caused; some emphasized that the method encouraged women's dependence on authority figures who imposed upon them complex and ritualistic routines; and some presented case histories that demonstrated the dangers of the Read method in women with personality disturbances.[44] Most significantly, like nineteenth-century physicians and clergymen who had objected to the use of ether or chloroform in labor because these agents were also used to induce pleasurable sensations (and this was viewed as unseemly and immoral for women in childbirth), Natural Childbirth critics made the quest for pleasure in childbirth suspect. Moreover, as will be described in more detail later, the "happy" pregnant woman was herself suspect since there were so many psychic conflicts that attended childbearing.[45]

Accordingly, critics of Natural Childbirth and advocates of pain-relieving drugs indicated their support of good or "better" obstetric anesthesia and analgesia. Specifically, they emphasized that good obstetric anesthesia and analgesia— meaning drugs that were safely and skillfully administered— was better than *no* pharmacologic pain relief at all. These physicians noted that although a delivery could be accomplished without drugs, both the woman and infant benefited from having received them.[46]

Advocates of drug use attempted to show that Natural Childbirth was less safe and more dangerous than childbirth controlled with drugs and also that controlled childbirth incorporated all of the best features of Natural Childbirth. With the refinement of regional block anesthesia techniques, such as caudal anesthesia, after World War II (techniques that allowed a woman to remain conscious but removed sensation of birth-giving), advocates of drug use emphasized that a woman could have an absolutely safe and painless delivery *and* still be awake, aware, fully conscious, and an active participant in the birth process.[47] Clifford B. Lull and Robert A. Hingson stated that the "advent of continuous caudal analgesia has opened up new fields in the *psychology* of childbirth" (italics mine). Applauding the fact that women who had caudals could hear their babies' first cry, they also stated that "this technic has returned to womanhood the heritage which she had to sacrifice through the use of various forms of anesthesia and amnesia."[48]

While some physicians believed that the "key" to pain relief in labor was to reduce women's fear of it, they and others also believed that the "key-hole whereby the entire problem of pain in childbirth may be unlocked is the sacral hiatus," a reference to the caudal technique.[49] Indeed, "the malleable caudal needle is the key [and] the adequate dosage of metycaine necessary to block the pathways of pain in parturition is the combination of that lock."[50] Like Twilight Sleep advocates, many physicians believed that a technique, such as caudal analgesia, could favorably alter the psychology of the childbearing woman and accomplish this more dependably than a method, such as Natural Childbirth, *which was itself psychological.*[51] For drug advocates, the skilled physician was the one who used psychology to prepare a woman to receive drugs and then selected the drug regimen most suited to her individual psychology.

Most significantly, for drug advocates, the "educated" patient (as Natural Childbirth patients were preferably called) was not necessarily the one who had been taught how to avoid drugs and instruments in childbirth, but rather she was the one who understood how desirable they could be.[52] The "fearless" patient (as Natural Childbirth patients were preferably called) was not necessarily the one who did not fear childbirth without drugs, but rather the one who did not fear childbirth with drugs. The "prepared" patient (as Natural Childbirth patients were preferably called) was not necessarily the one who had been trained to rely on her own resources in labor to combat pain, but rather she was the one who had been prepared during pregnancy and early labor (in part with preanesthetic drugs) to receive drugs in the later stages of labor. By emphasizing such factors and using such trigger words as consciousness, fearlessness, participation, and satisfaction, drug advocates demonstrated their incorporation of some of the language and goals of Natural Childbirth at the same time that they rejected the philosophy on which the method was based and its central goal, namely, to feel childbirth and to master it without artificial aid. In effect, drug advocates successfully "colonialized" Natural Childbirth and assimilated it into prophylactic obstetrics.[53]

Notes

1. Francis Holmes, "Psychogenic Factors in Obstetrics," *California and Western Medicine* 63 (October 1945):162; Report of the Com-

mittee on Infancy and Early Childhood of the American Society for Research on Psychosomatic Problems," *Psychosomatic Medicine* 7 (July 1945):224–34; Howard C. Walser, "Fear, An Important Etiological Factor in Obstetric Problems," *American Journal of Obstetrics and Gynecology* 55 (May 1948):799–805; and Edward Weiss and O. Spurgeon English, *Psychosomatic Medicine: The Clinical Application of Psychopathology to General Medical Problems* (Philadelphia: W. B. Saunders, 1943), p. 614.

2. In general American usage, Grantly Dick-Read is referred to as Read, not as Dick-Read. In addition, when "Natural Childbirth" appears in capital letters, it refers to Read's theory and method as he presented it and as Americans interpreted it. In the 1940s and 1950s, Natural Childbirth was the Read method and no other.

3. Read's ideas may be found in Grantly Dick-Read, *Childbirth Without Fear: The Principles and Practice of Natural Childbirth* (New York: Harper and Brothers, 1944). There are also a number of paperback versions of this text that were either written exclusively by Read or include excerpts of many of Read's works along with material written by others. Two such versions used for this study are *Childbirth Without Fear: The Principles and Practice of Natural Childbirth*, 2nd ed., rev. (New York: Harper and Row, Har/Row Books, 1970) and *Childbirth Without Fear*, 4th ed., rev., ed. Helen Wessel and Harlan F. Ellis (New York: Harper and Row, Perennial Library, 1979). See also Grantly Dick-Read's *Birth of a Child* (New York: Vanguard Press, 1950); *Introduction to Motherhood* (New York: Harper and Brothers, 1950); *The Natural Childbirth Primer* (New York: Harper and Brothers, 1955); and *No Time for Fear* (New York: Harper and Brothers, 1955).

4. Gretta Palmer, "Having your Baby the New Way," *Collier's*, 13 November 1948, pp. 26–27, clipping in Thoms' scrapbooks, Yale Medical History Library, New Haven, Conn.

5. Blackwell Sawyer, "Experiences With the Labor Procedure of Grantly Dick-Read," *American Journal of Obstetrics and Gynecology* 51 (June 1946):852–58.

6. *Childbirth Without Fear*, 4th ed., p. 291.

7. Joseph B. DeLee, *The Principles and Practice of Obstetrics*, 7th ed. (Philadelphia: W. B. Saunders, 1938), pp. 339–40. Recall that DeLee lamented the need for medical intervention in childbirth with drugs and instruments and regretted the abuse of prophylactic obstetrics. Accordingly, he was willing to allow that Read's ideas might have some merit and could help to reduce intervention in childbirth. Read was pleased with DeLee's apparent support. Ironically, DeLee, who spent much of his career warning women and professionals of

the dangers of natural birth, was credited as being one of the first physicians to "promote the idea that labor is naturally painless, and should be a normal and pleasurable experience." This citation, in William S. Kroger and S. Charles Freed, *Psychosomatic Gynecology: Including Problems of Obstetrical Care* (Philadelphia: W. B. Saunders, 1951), p. 123, suggests that some American physicians simply could not allow that Read had invented anything new. American physicians' ambivalence about the Read method will be described in more detail in the chapters 4, 5, and 6.

8. Paul De Kruif, "Why Should Mothers Die?" *Ladies Home Journal*, March 1936, p. 101. This is the first article in the series.

9. *Childbirth Without Fear*, 4th ed., p. 301.

10. Janet Andrews, "Taking the Fear Out of Childbirth," *Parents Magazine*, May 1943, pp. 30–31, 99; H. Bundeson, "The Needless Fear of Childbirth," *Ladies Home Journal*, November 1944, pp. 61, 129.

11. Grantly Dick-Read to Herbert Thoms, 25 November 1954, private collection of Margaret Thoms. This remark should be understood as both Read's acknowledgment that Natural Childbirth was not a completely revolutionary idea *and* as an appeal to Thoms and the world that he be viewed as the originator of Natural Childbirth. From Read's writings, his letters to Thoms, as well as from Noyes Thomas' biography of Read, *Doctor Courageous: The Story of Dr. Grantly Dick-Read* (Melbourne: William Heinemann Ltd., 1957), it is clear that Read was both saddened and angered by the British medical community's rejection of him and his ideas and by the opposition he encountered from American physicians, especially their tendency to dismiss his method as unscientific or nothing new. Read clearly wanted his method to be accepted to the point where it would no longer seem new, but also he wanted the recognition that any revolutionary thinker should receive. Consequently, the cited remark is infused with ambivalent feelings.

12. Alice B. Stockham, *Tokology: A Book For Every Woman*, 3rd ed. (New York: R. F. Fenno, 1911).

13. Clifford B. Lull and Robert A. Hingson, *Control of Pain in Childbirth: Anesthesia, Analgesia, Amnesia* (Philadelphia: J. B. Lippincott, 1944), pp. 114–15; C. O. McCormick, "Rectal Ether Analgesia in Obstetrics," *American Journal of Nursing* 33 (May 1933):419.

14. Grantly Dick-Read to Herbert Thoms, 1 March 1949, private collection of Margaret Thoms.

15. Annual Report, 1918–1958, p. 13, files of the Maternity Center Association of New York, New York City.

16. As Eugene Declercq, in "Painless Childbirth in America: The Impact of Culture, Technology and Feminism on Childbearing," in-

dicates, some nineteenth-century physicians also employed rapid breathing techniques. He cites an 1880 *Philadelphia Medical Times* article. I thank Dr. Declercq for sharing this unpublished paper.

17. "Natural or Unnatural?" *Time*, 19 January 1953, p. 52.

18. Annual Report, 1948, Maternity Center files.

19. Palmer, "Having Your Baby," pp. 26–27, 61. This account of how Yale physicians became involved in Natural Childbirth is essentially corroborated by Thoms and Goodrich who attributed their involvement to women's interest. See, for example, the introduction to Herbert Thoms, *Training for Childbirth: A Program of Natural Childbirth With Rooming-In* (New York: McGraw-Hill, 1950).

20. Leon Chertok, *Psychosomatic Methods in Painless Childbirth: History, Theory and Practice*, trans. Denis Leigh (New York: Pergamon Press, 1959), p. 64; "Natural Childbirth Without Pain," *New Haven Register*, 2 March 1947, p. 2, clipping in Thoms' scrapbooks.

21. See the log for 1947, Maternity Center files.

22. Grantly Dick-Read to Herbert Thoms, 22 January 1947 and 13 February 1947, private collection of Margaret Thoms.

23. Thoms, *Training*; Herbert Thoms with L. Roth, *Understanding Natural Childbirth: A Book for the Expectant Mother* (New York: McGraw-Hill, 1950). See also Edith Jackson, "New Trends in Maternity Care," *American Journal of Nursing* 55 (May 1955):84–87. As physician director of Yale's rooming-in program, she described Yale's initiative in incorporating the psychosomatic approach into maternity care as does "Natural Childbirth Without Pain," *New Haven Register*, p. 3.

24. Frederick W. Goodrich and Herbert Thoms, "A Clinical Study of Natural Childbirth: A Preliminary Report from a Teaching Ward Service," *American Journal of Obstetrics and Gynecology* 56 (November 1948):875–83.

25. Two of the four Thoms scrapbooks are filled with newspaper and magazine clippings dating from the beginning of the Yale program.

26. See the footnote on p. 301 of *Childbirth Without Fear*, 4th ed. An attempt was made to obtain sales figures from the publisher, but these were discarded.

27. "The Story of the Work of the Maternity Center Association for the Families of America, 1946–51," Maternity Center files. The logs of the association; articles in *Briefs*, its periodical publication; and lay publications on the method also reflect interest in it.

28. Horace T. Gardner to Herbert Thoms, 4 April 1950, private collection of Margaret Thoms.

29. Ann Lindsay to Herbert Thoms, 14 February 1952, private collection of Margaret Thoms.

30. See the remarks on p. 125 following Frederick W. Goodrich, "Experience With Natural Childbirth," *Public Health Nursing* 41 (March 1949).

31. B. M. McKinney, "The Pleasure of Childbirth," *Ladies Home Journal*, April 1949, pp. 116, 118–20.

32. "Natural Childbirth," *Life*, 30 January 1950, p. 71.

33. Duncan E. Reid and Mandel E. Cohen, "Evaluation of Present Day Trends in Obstetrics," *Journal of the American Medical Association*, 4 March 1950, pp. 615–22.

34. Nicholson J. Eastman, "The Multi-Disciplinary Approach to Obstetrics," *Bulletin of Maternal Welfare* 4 (May-June 1957):16–22; Margaret Mead, *Male and Female* (New York: William Morrow, 1949), p. 376. The term *artifices* is Eastman's.

35. Lawrence E. Arnold, "Analgesia in Obstetrics: An Analysis of 500 Consecutive Cases," *Texas State Journal of Medicine* 37 (July 1941):211–15; Frederick H. Falls, "The Present Status of Pain Relief in Labor," *Kentucky Medical Journal* 43 (February 1945):48–52; J. C. Furnas, "What Price Pain," *Ladies Home Journal*, February 1940, p. 24; Charles Gould and B. C. Hirst, "Current Technics for Obstetric Analgesia and Anesthesia," *American Journal of Obstetrics and Gynecology* 30 (August 1935):257–63; Arthur T. Shimer, "Obstetric Analgesia and Anesthesia: What is the Price for Relief of Pain?" *Bulletin of Maternal Welfare* 5 (May-June 1958):18–20; Franklin F. Snyder, *Obstetric Analgesia and Anesthesia: Their Effects Upon Labor and the Child* (Philadelphia: W. B. Saunders, 1949), p. v; and Charles E. Stevenson, "Maternal Deaths from Obstetric Anesthesia and Analgesia: Can They Be Eliminated?" *Obstetrics and Gynecology* 8 (July 1956):88.

36. Hermann S. Rhujr, "Obstetric Anesthesia," *Obstetrics and Gynecology* 11 (June 1958):728.

37. Following is an alphabetical listing of relevant reports. Committee on Maternal Mortality, "Analysis of Causes of Maternal Deaths in Massachusetts During 1941, Anesthesia," *New England Journal of Medicine* 7 (January 1943):36–37; William A. Cull and Robert A. Hingson, "Dedication, Education, and Organization in the Round-The-Clock Staffing of a Modern Obstetrical Analgesia and Anesthesia Service," *Bulletin of Maternal Welfare* 4 (September-October 1957):17–26; M. Edward Davis and Thomas G. Gready, "A Review of the Maternal Mortality at the Chicago Lying-In Hospital, 1931–1945," *American Journal of Obstetrics and Gynecology* 51 (March 1946):492–

513; J. E. Fitzgerald and Augusta Webster, "Nineteen-Year Survey of Maternal Mortality at the Cook County Hospital," *American Journal of Obstetrics and Gynecology* 65 (March 1953):528–33; Edwin M. Gold and Helen M. Wallace, "A Study of Maternal Deaths in New York City for 1947," *New York State Journal of Medicine*, 15 July 1949, pp. 1676–80; L. M. Hellman and Robert A. Hingson, "Some Modern Aspects of Anesthesia and Analgesia," *New York State Journal of Medicine*, 15 July 1952, pp. 1770–73; James R. Herron, "Anesthesia in Obstetrics—Killer!" *Bulletin of Maternal Welfare* 3 (March-April 1956):9–12; Robert A. Hingson and Louis M. Hellman, "Organization of Obstetric Anesthesia on a Twenty-Four Hour Basis in a Large and a Small Hospital," *Anesthesiology* 12 (November 1951):745–52; Milton D. Klein et al., "Maternal Deaths Caused by Anesthesia in the Borough of the Bronx from 1940 to 1951," *New York State Journal of Medicine*, 1 December 1953, pp. 2861–66; Frank R. Lock and Frank C. Geiss, "The Anesthetic Hazards in Obstetrics," *American Journal of Obstetrics and Gynecology* 70 (October 1955):861–75; Ruth B. Merrill and Robert A. Hingson, "Study of Incidence of Maternal Mortality from Aspiration of Vomitus During Anesthesia in Major Obstetric Hospitals in the United States," *Current Researches in Anesthesia and Analgesia* 30 (May-June 1951):121–35; Robert McNair Mitchell, "Maternal Mortality in the Pennsylvania Hospital (Philadelphia Lying-In Hospital): Tabular Review of Maternal Deaths, 1929–1953," *Obstetrics and Gynecology* 5 (February 1955):123–36; Harrold A. Ott and Mary Lou Boyd, "Michigan Mortality Study 1950–1952, Category V. Anesthesia," *Journal of the Michigan State Medical Society* 54 (February 1955):182–84; Otto C. Phillips, "The Role of Anesthesia in Obstetric Mortality: A Review of 455,553 Live Births from 1936 to 1958 in the City of Baltimore," *Current Researches in Anesthesia and Analgesia* 40 (September-October 1961):557–66; and Robert A. Ross, "Maternal Mortality: Omissions and Commissions," *Virginia Medical Monthly* 83 (February 1956):45–47.

38. The following citations represent all of the investigative reports on Natural Childbirth found in American professional literature between 1946 and 1960 and written by physicians and others practicing in American hospitals. Canadian studies were not considered. The citations are listed in order of appearance (instead of alphabetically by the author's last name) since data from an earlier study by an investigator or group of investigators were sometimes included in reports of later studies. In addition, studies tended to be reviewed in other articles that did not contain original investigative material. For example, C. Lee Buxton's "Prepared Childbirth and Rooming-In at Yale," *The Pennsylvania Medical Journal* 60 (Febru-

ary 1957):171–76, contains a review of the 1954 study by Thoms and Karlovsky, which will be cited here. In short, few studies on Natural Childbirth attempted to quantify outcomes or explain outcomes in a systematic fashion in comparison with the volume of investigative reports on pain-relieving drugs in childbirth. Sawyer, "Experiences with the Labor Procedure"; Goodrich and Thoms, "Clinical Study of Natural Childbirth"; Laurence G. Roth, "Natural Childbirth in a General Hospital," *American Journal of Obstetrics and Gynecology* 61 (January 1951):167–72; Herbert Thoms and Robert H. Wyatt, "One Thousand Consecutive Deliveries Under a Training for Childbirth Program," *American Journal of Obstetrics and Gynecology* 61 (January 1951):205–9; John E. Stoll, "Experiences with Natural Childbirth: Report of Two Hundred Cases from Private Practice and Public Clinic, Including Four Sets of Twins," *The Western Journal of Surgery, Obstetrics and Gynecology* 59 (February 1951):49–55; Harold B. Davidson, "Education for Childbirth: A Preliminary Report," *New York Medicine*, 20 April 1952, pp. 16–21, 34–40; H. Lloyd Miller, Francis E. Flannery, and Dorothy Bell, "Education for Childbirth in Private Practice: 450 Consecutive Cases," *American Journal of Obstetrics and Gynecology* 63 (April 1952):792–99; H. Lloyd Miller and Francis E. Flannery, "Education for Childbirth in Private Practice (669 Consecutive Cases)," *Journal of Iowa State Medical Society* 43 (January 1953):9–14. This includes the 450 cases previously reported (above) by these investigators; William B. D. Van Auken and David R. Tomlinson, "An Appraisal of Patient Training for Childbirth," *American Journal of Obstetrics and Gynecology* 66 (July 1953):100–4; Harold B. Davidson, "The Psychosomatic Aspects of Educated Childbirth," *New York State Journal of Medicine*, 1 November 1953, pp. 2499–2503; Herbert Thoms and Emil D. Karlovsky, "Two Thousand Deliveries Under a Training for Childbirth Program: A Statistical Survey and Commentary," *American Journal of Obstetrics and Gynecology* 68 (July 1954):279–84. This includes the one thousand deliveries Thoms and Wyatt studied in 1951; Marion D. Laird and Margaret Hogan, "An Elective Program on Preparation for Childbirth at the Sloane Hospital For Women, May 1951, to June 1953," *American Journal of Obstetrics and Gynecology* 72 (September 1956):641–47; H. L. Miller, "Education for Childbirth: A Report of 3177 Consecutive Deliveries in Private Practice," *Medical Times* 86 (April 1958):464–72. This includes the 669 cases studied in 1953; and Fred D. Kartchner, "Active Participation in Childbirth: A Psychosomatic Approach to Pregnancy and Parturition," *American Journal of Obstetrics and Gynecology* 75 (June 1958):1244–53.

39. In addition to the formal studies lisited in note 38, see Joan

Beck, "Why Young Mothers Feel Cheated," *Bulletin of Maternal Welfare* 5 (January-February 1958):20–23; Hazel Corbin, "Natural Childbirth," *American Journal of Nursing* 49 (October 1949):660–62; Julie Harris, as told to Betty Friedan, "I Was Afraid to Have a Baby," *McCall's*, December 1956, pp. 68–74; J. H. Pollack, "The Case for Natural Childbirth," *Cosmopolitan*, July 1953, pp. 39–43; Herbert Thoms and Ernestine Wiedenbach, "Support During Labor: Outline of Practice and Summary of Results from the Mother's Viewpoint," *Journal of the American Medical Association*, 4 September 1954, pp. 3–5; and Ernestine Wiedenbach, "Childbirth as Mothers Say They Like It," *Public Health Nursing* 41 (August 1949):417–21. Wiedenbach was a key nursing figure in the Natural Childbirth movement.

40. Cull and Hingson, "Dedication, Education, and Organization," p. 19; Charles A. Gordon, Alexander H. Rosenthal, and James L. O'Leary, "Anesthesia," *American Journal of Surgery* 81 (February 1951):238; and Reid and Cohen, "Evaluation of Present Day Trends," pp. 615–22. Reid and Cohen suggested that the reason the maternal mortality rate was higher in the black population than in the white was because black women had more "natural" births, meaning births without medical intervention. Yet there is conflicting evidence on the extent to which nonwhite women had "natural" births as opposed to births controlled by drugs and instruments. On the one hand, there was still a belief that white, upper-class women needed more assistance at birth, thus making them more subject to operative intervention. Besides, they were in a position to *pay* for this kind of childbirth. In addition, upper-class women did constitute the majority of women giving birth in hospitals through the 1940s and were thus more likely to be "assisted" than women who gave birth at home. On the other hand, physicians did experiment with or practice new medical techniques on "charity" or "ward" patients, suggesting that poor women, among them many nonwhite women, were more subject to obstetric intervention.

41. See the discussion following Arthur Bill, "Analgesia and Anesthesia and Their Bearing Upon the Problem of Shortened Labor," *American Journal of Obstetrics and Gynecology* 34 (November 1937):879; Mary R. Lester and Leroy W. Krumperman, "Anesthesia and Analgesia," *Clinical Obstetrics and Gynecology* 1 (December 1958):977.

42. "Death Rise Feared in 'Natural' Births," *New York Times*, 12 November 1949, p. 18.

43. " 'Natural Childbirth' Program Oversold, Says U.S. Expert," *New Haven Journal-Courier*, 17 November 1950, p. 10, clipping in Thoms' scrapbooks.

44. Arthur J. Mandy et al., "Is Natural Childbirth Natural?" *Psychosomatic Medicine* 14 (November-December 1952):431–38; Floyd Sterling Rogers, "Dangers of the Read Method in Patients With Major Personality Problems," *American Journal of Obstetrics and Gynecology* 71 (June 1956):1236–41.

45. Walter Channing, *A Treatise on Etherization in Childbirth* (Boston: William D. Ticknor, 1848), pp. 135–58; Robert N. Crendick, "The Patient Psychologically Unprepared for Labor," *Clinical Obstetrics and Gynecology* 2 (June 1959):318; and Harold Speert, *Obstetrics and Gynecology in America: A History* (Chicago: American College of Obstetricians and Gynecologists, 1980), p. 137. Physicians' and dentists' observations of the effects of agents such as ether on participants in ether frolics, a popular early nineteenth-century form of entertainment, helped lead to the use of them for pain relief.

46. Rhujr, "Obstetric Anesthesia," p. 728; Carl T. Javert and James D. Hardy, "Influence of Analgesics on Pain Intensity During Labor (With a Note on 'Natural Childbirth')," *Anesthesiology* 12 (March 1951):211. According to Javert and Hardy, the greater efficiency of labor achieved with analgesic drugs correctly given "justifies" their use in "healthy women."

47. John J. Bonica, "Obstetric Analgesia and Anesthesia in General Practice," *Journal of the American Medical Association*, 28 December 1957, p. 2152.

48. Lull and Hingson, *Control of Pain*, p. 115.

49. Falls, "Present Status of Pain Relief," p. 52.

50. Waldo B. Edwards and Robert A. Hingson, "The Present Status of Continuous Caudal Analgesia in Obstetrics," *Bulletin of the New York Academy of Medicine* 19 (July 1943):514.

51. For example, Lester and Krumperman, "Anesthesia and Analgesia," indicated on p. 978 how effective barbiturates were, not against "real" pain but against anxiety. Nicholson Eastman, in "The Middle Road in Obstetrics," *Ladies Home Journal*, May 1952, p. 11, stated that Natural Childbirth was not a "dependable" substitute for obstetric anesthesia and analgesia.

52. Most Americans and Read himself were uncomfortable with the term "natural" to describe the Read method, since it led to so many misconceptions.

53. Ann Oakley, in "A Case of Maternity: Paradigms of Women as Maternity Cases," *Signs: Journal of Women in Culture and Society* 4 (Summer 1979):629, used the word "colonized" in a similar context.

THE QUEST FOR PLEASURE: THE AMERICANIZATION OF NATURAL CHILDBIRTH _____

The debate about whether it was better or worse for women in labor to receive pain-relieving drugs revealed the extent to which Grantly Dick-Read's theory and method of Natural Childbirth were altered to fit the prevailing American conception of what childbirth was like and how it should be conducted. Indeed, there existed skepticism and criticism of Natural Childbirth, but there was never really any clear line between advocacy of Natural Childbirth and advocacy of drug use. Americans, it seems, thought it more prudent and less "extreme" to pursue a "middle road" in matters relating to the care of childbearing women.[1] Some modifications of the Read method were necessary because of the types and numbers of personnel, services, and facilities available in the United States for maternity care, and some were warranted by Americans' actual experiences with the method.

Read had envisioned that Natural Childbirth would be practiced in an environment physically and psychologically conducive to its successful use by the laboring women. In such an environment, a woman labored in privacy, perhaps with her husband, but she was never left alone without the sympathetic and competent assistance of either her midwife or her physician—both of whom fervently believed in the normality and natural painlessness of childbirth.

Yet several features of American maternity care persistently intruded on this vision. Specifically, neither the average physician who attended women in labor nor the obstetric nurse were really prepared by education or training or were in a position to conduct childbirth as if it were a normal and painless event. Physicians and nurses were not ready to relinquish all of those routines of care that they sincerely believed had contributed to the dramatic improvement in maternal and infant health over the first half of the twentieth century. These routines included such "prophylactic" measures as the administration of intravenous fluids to prevent dehydration and to keep the laboring woman prepared to receive any pain-relieving drugs she might require; the use of enemas and perineal shaves to prevent contamination of the delivery site and to prepare the woman for any operative intervention she might require; and the use of forceps and episiotomy to prevent perineal trauma and injury to the fetus. Moreover, as described previously, professionals had become used to and skilled in caring for women under the influence of drugs, namely women who were semiconscious or unconscious or thrashing about. Having made the choice to practice prophylactic obstetrics, having invested time and energy in mastering its techniques, and, most importantly, having accepted the idea that "natural" labor was potentially dangerous in a time when large numbers of women were injured and died in childbirth, professionals found it difficult to alter their practice and the philosophy on which it was based.

Furthermore, the very physical environment of the typical American labor and delivery suite was very different from the kind of setting deemed important to the success of the Read method. Most American women were having their babies in hospitals by the end of the 1940s, and hospitals, intended to treat the sick, were not designed to satisfy the needs of maternity patients. Women frequently labored in rather starkly decorated, semiprivate or ward settings in which the sights, smells, and sounds of one woman's labor could easily influence the labor progress of another and in which there were constant visual reminders of the possibility that labor might not proceed naturally or painlessly. Nurses' and physicians' costumes reminded women of the possibility of infection; medication administration equipment reminded them that they might need to have drugs; and the delivery room itself suggested the imminent possibility of operative intervention. In effect, the environment of the laboring woman—its strangeness and the fear this strangeness engendered in her—made it even more likely that she would require drugs and instruments to master labor.

The practice of rotating nurses and house physicians two to three times over a twenty-four-hour period made it very difficult for the professional attendant and the laboring woman to establish the close personal relationship considered crucial to the success of Natural Childbirth. Finally, there were simply not enough physicians or nurses available in the country as a whole, especially in the era of the baby boom, to provide every woman with the exclusive services of one nurse and one doctor for the duration of her labor. Natural Childbirth was perceived as a method that demanded more time and work from already overtaxed caregivers. Moreover, it demanded a renewed intimacy with a patient who was now conscious of her surroundings. In short, even if the majority of Americans, physicians, nurses, and the general public had agreed with every aspect of Read's theory and method, they would still have found it incredibly hard to implement Natural Childbirth given the typical circumstances and milieu in which women gave birth.

Even advocates of the Read method could not agree with Read's basic assumption that normal labor was painless. For example, Goodrich, in his 1949 report on the Yale program, noted that only 2 percent of four hundred women studied had found labor to be painless.[2] Thoms and Karlovsky, in their 1954 report on two thousand women who had participated in the Yale program, noted that 62 percent of these women had required small doses of either Demerol or Seconal, and 66 percent had required intermittent second-stage anesthesia with Trilene or nitrous oxide. Only 34 percent of these women had required no analgesia in the first stage, and only 29 percent had required no anesthesia in the second stage.[3] Laird and

Hogan, in their 1956 report on women in a Natural Childbirth program in New York, also indicated that most of them needed at least minimal doses of pain-relieving drugs.[4]

Advocates of Natural Childbirth insisted, therefore, that it was deceptive to promise women painless births and warned of the possible emotional damage to women who chose the method and were then inadvertently made to feel like failures if they required drugs.[5] Most significantly, both advocates and critics of Natural Childbirth viewed the use of drugs as the last resort for women anxious about or in pain. Advocates were forced to defend the method against the commonly held belief that physicians practicing it deliberately withheld drugs from women by emphasizing that drugs were always available to anyone who needed them. Moreover, where the medical imperative used to be proving the superiority of drugs and instruments over "natural" birth, the new imperative was proving that Natural Childbirth was superior to drugs and instruments, using criteria more appropriate to evaluating drugs and instruments.[6]

In stating their continued reliance on drugs both to help women cope with pain and *to help them succeed with Natural Childbirth*, advocates demonstrated that they really agreed with Natural Childbirth critics that drugs were ultimately the most dependable measures against pain in the majority of women. Most Americans on either side of the Natural Childbirth argument agreed with each other, in direct contrast to Read's belief, that labor was painful even if a woman was not afraid of it. In fact, most American publications concerning the method revealed that no pain was not what women experienced, but rather less pain or a more positive attitude toward pain, and that no drugs was not what was required, but rather lesser amounts of drugs. The difference between Natural Childbirth and childbirth controlled with drugs became for Americans essentially one of degree not of kind.

Accordingly, the major argument developed by advocates did not concern the painlessness of childbirth per se but rather the pleasure women could derive from the method in comparison with the satisfaction anyone would experience in childbirth from obtaining mere pain relief with any drug regimen. Natural

Childbirth advocates increasingly stressed that the primary goal of the method was not the alleviation of pain nor even the avoidance of drugs per se but rather the maximization of pleasure. American advocates deemphasized Read's strong feelings against obstetric management of childbirth with artificial aids and underscored his equally strong feelings concerning the satisfaction possible in childbirth.

A *New York Herald Tribune* article indicated that the aim of the Yale program was not painlessness but rather the enhancement of a woman's sense of pleasure and achievement.[7] A *West Hartford News* feature noted that Read emphasized fear as the "enemy" of women in labor, but Herbert Thoms emphasized joy as their "ally."[8] Thoms had stated that too much emphasis was placed on "conscious" and "spontaneous" birth, suggesting that a woman could be happy even if asleep at the birth of her child or in need of operative assistance.[9] He and Yale psychologist Lawrence Freedman observed that the Yale program sought neither "naturalness" and "painlessness" nor "consciousness" and the elimination of pain-relieving drugs but rather a "subjectively happy" patient and a "medically satisfactory" pregnancy and labor.[10] Reports on the Yale program indicated that the criteria for operative assistance in childbirth had not changed in the execution of Natural Childbirth, and Read himself commented to Thoms how their practice of childbirth differed from one another, including the use of stirrups and episiotomy.[11]

The Maternity Center Association and Nicholson Eastman urged Americans to dismiss the notion that Natural Childbirth was a "competitor of medical analgesics and anesthetics" since Natural Childbirth *included* the judicious use of pain-relieving drugs.[12] A magazine article favoring the method indicated that it was a "myth" that it excluded drugs.[13] Finally, Vera Keane, an important nurse advocate of the method, declared that the "yardsticks of success" in childbirth were not the length of labor, the amount of medications used, nor the conduct of labor itself, but rather the satisfaction of the patient.[14] Most importantly, Americans' conception of Natural Childbirth was sometimes virtually indistinguishable from their view of childbirth with drugs. Natural or educated or prepared childbirth might conceivably include any routine or technique, with the exception of cesarean section, deemed necessary by the physician and might conceivably exclude any part of the Read program deemed unnecessary by him—so long as a *happy* patient was the end result. Investigative reports on Natural Childbirth reveal wide variations in antepartum training (from little to all of Read's educative and exercise components) and intrapartal support (from none to constant professional attendance and encouragement).[15]

While Read had envisioned Natural Childbirth for any woman provided she had no medical or obstetric complications, advocates as well as critics saw it as suitable for only a select few, that is, not "universally applicable," implying that childbirth with drugs was still the best choice for the majority of women.[16] Some advocates also harbored suspicions about the types of women attracted to the method and about its impact on their mental health; others suggested that only intelligent and motivated women could succeed with the method; and still others actually limited the numbers of women who might have chosen it by never suggesting it to any of their patients until they themselves mentioned it "spontaneously."[17] In the apparent effort to find the women who would most likely succeed with it and thus place it in a favorable light, advocates themselves inadvertently ensured that the method would not have the mass appeal of drugs.

More precisely, childbirth controlled with drugs was the norm, and any laboring woman was perceived as eligible to receive them. There was no such thing as candidacy for drug use. While a single drug or drug regimen might be contraindicated in a particular case, there was no labor patient for whom some drug could not be found. If a woman could not have general anesthesia, she could have spinal. If she could not have morphine, she could have Demerol.[18] Moreover, no woman had to ask to receive drugs. Although physicians depicted childbirth controlled with drugs as something women *chose* to have (a partial truth), by the 1930s, drugs were a matter of course, an integral part of the routine practice of obstetrics and, most importantly, out of the realm of choice for women. A woman would have had to ask *not* to receive drugs.[19]

In contrast, for a woman to be eligible for Natural Childbirth, she had to be a good "candidate." For example, she had to be judged by a physician as normal, obstetrically, medically, and psychologically. Moreover, a woman, in many cases (if not most), had to ask for Natural Childbirth, and that meant she had to know about it beforehand. While both "private" and "ward" or "staff" patients participated in Natural Childbirth programs, the private patient was more likely to have asked for the method herself, and the ward patient was more likely to be dependent on her caregivers to tell her about it and offer it to her. In addition, if the ward patient chose Natural Childbirth, she was also very likely to have to practice and execute it with little professional support.[20]

Both critics and advocates of the method frowned on *imposing* it on women or placing them under its influence. Natural Childbirth proponents resisted the method's association with hypnosis because hypnosis was depicted as unscientific and cultic and almost like brainwashing. The routine use of pain-relieving drugs and instruments was not viewed as an imposition even though women now had little choice concerning their use.[21]

In short, while critics of Natural Childbirth assimilated it into prevailing obstetric practice, advocates also compromised it. Even allowing for the many obstacles that the method faced in the typical American labor setting, the method was neither interpreted nor practiced uniformly. Most significantly, advocates were never really convinced that Natural Childbirth, unless modified, could ever be anything more than an alternative for some women to childbirth controlled with drugs. Both advocates and critics of Natural Childbirth traveled the middle road—advocates paying due homage to the importance of pain-relieving drugs and critics paying due homage to the importance of satisfaction.

Natural Childbirth, the Feminine Mystique, and Freud

No matter how Americans actually practiced Natural Childbirth, it seemed to make women more pleased with themselves as women. One woman stated how "important" she felt knowing that she was attending the only school of its kind in the United States (the Yale program).[22] A *Modern Romances* article described the "ideal Read-method mother" as the rather average woman who went to work instead of to college, married young, started her family early, and was no stranger to scrubbing brushes and wash tubs.[23] The author of this article suggested how women became unaverage when they chose Natural Childbirth. Another journalist depicted the method as one that only bright women could successfully use, and Frederick W. Goodrich commented on how "triumphant" the Natural Childbirth patient felt because she "knew that she had helped to have her baby."[24]

As depicted by proponents of Natural Childbirth, the woman who chose it was the center of attention in the delivery room and not the "necessary evil" she used to be.[25] Like the Twilight Sleep mother before her, the Read mother was viewed as an adventurer charting a new course that other women could follow. She was a heroine who inspired awe in those who witnessed her achievement. Natural Childbirth made the ordinary woman extraordinary. Natural Childbirth promised that a woman would no longer be cheated of the greatest event in her life. Most importantly, Natural Childbirth promised happiness, fulfillment, pride, and a sense of self-esteem to women in an era when maternity was the best and really only acceptable source of them.

Informed by the feminine mystique, with its emphasis on the home, family, and motherhood, Natural Childbirth served to highlight the extent to which a woman's happiness in childbirth was vital, not only to herself but also to the harmony of the family. Natural Childbirth emphasized a woman's pleasure in childbirth as her right and as the secure foundation on which the happiness of the family and society rested. In war or in peace, women had to be willing to give birth, at least several times, and Natural Childbirth advocates underscored not only how much ecstasy the experience might involve but also how much education, preparation, and training giving birth required. Indeed, some observers of women were concerned that modern education was diverting women away from their biological "urge" to reproduce, creating in the process untold "emotional stress" and engendering dangerous competition in the workplace between women and men.[26] Others showed that Natural Childbirth reeducated and retrained women to view maternity as a full-time profession and their main purpose in life.[27]

Although most physicians believed that the method could never replace drugs as pain-relieving measures, they did believe that Natural Childbirth's most positive feature was its apparent ability to make childbirth "attractive and more gratifying" to women.[28] In fact, some observers implied that Natural Childbirth not only made women happier giving birth but it also made them happier with the hospital care they were already receiving.[29] In short, the rhetoric of Natural Childbirth reinforced the ideology of the feminine mystique and prophylactic obstetrics. The method was intended to offset the negative aspects of drug and instrument use and hospital care, not to replace them. The method was intended to reinforce women's desire to bear children, not to divert them from it. The method was intended to make everyone—women and their caregivers—happier. Natural Childbirth meant "the happy way to have a baby."[30]

While Natural Childbirth promised the most happiness in the childbirth experience, virtually everyone agreed that the key variable affecting happiness was not any specific method of childbirth but rather the quality of the physician-patient relationship. Several studies demonstrated that behind every happy maternity patient, whether under the influence of drugs or Natural Childbirth, was a doctor in whom she had placed her faith and her fate.[31] Indeed, Read himself had criticized his medical colleagues for their undue reliance on "man's contrivances" instead of the "Creator's devices" in the management of childbirth; nevertheless, he viewed physicians as the most important determinants of the success or failure of Natural Childbirth.[32]

According to Read, the obstetrician had a mission in the postwar world. Far from forfeiting his important role as mentor to the woman who entered the "holy estate" of maternity,[33] the physician could redeem himself by offering her the joy of a natural birth and thus fulfill his worldly mission of creating a "new quality of man" through her.[34] While drugs and instruments had once solely legitimated the obstetrician's preeminent place in the care of the childbearing woman, Natural Childbirth, a method only he could properly offer her, was an even better justification for it. Still in control of obstetric technology but now armed with nature, the physician could humanize the birth experience. In fact, the physician who practiced Natural Childbirth made the "art of natural motherhood" more perfect by supervising and improving on the "original models from the great factories of human life."[35]

American physicians certainly did not object in the main to Read's favorable portrayal of the obstetrician since it was not substantively different from the way they saw themselves. Nineteenth-and early twentieth-century physicians also viewed themselves as the " 'perfecting agency' " of society through their ministrations to childbearing women.[36] In the same vein, the modern physician, committed to science and progress, carefully examined, weighed, measured, probed, and evaluated pregnant women, also for the greater good.[37]

Yet obstetricians and psychiatrists increasingly depicted the childbearing woman, the physician, and the relationship they shared with each other in a manner distinctively different from the way Read had. While Read saw the physician and patient in a mutually cooperative relationship (albeit with the physician in the dominant role), medical writers tended to depict a psychologically tenuous relationship fraught with libidinal tensions.

In contrast to Read's view that the fear of childbirth was an abnormal product of civilization, those physicians who expressed themselves on the subject in the 1940s and 1950s believed that it was a normal manifestation in a group of people whose normality was itself suspect. One physician posed the question for his medical colleagues in obstetrics-gynecology and psychiatry when he pondered whether the pregnant woman was or really ever had been a *normal* person.[38]

Indeed, many medical writers on the psychology of women agreed that it was especially difficult to separate normality from deviance in the childbearing woman since there were so many aspects of maternity that bordered on the pathological. They sympathized more readily with the ideas of Helene Deutsch who, unlike Read, suggested that physical or psychological deviations in childbirth derived primarily from women themselves, not civilization. Deutsch charged Read with having "too realistic" and, therefore, too superficial a view of the fear of childbirth, which she believed was profoundly rooted in every woman's psyche.[39] For Deutsch and her followers, neither Natural Childbirth by itself nor any other childbirth regimen could easily uproot the atavistic terror and anguish or the "pregnophobia" that existed in women whether they were pregnant or not.

Ernst Simmel, a distinguished emigré analyst, depicted the gynecologist as the "custodian of the female reproductive organ system, the normality of which guarantees normal wives, normal husbands, happy marriages, and normal children."[40] According to him, women were "beset" with certain "psychobiological" problems that tended toward "failures in the mental or physical development to mature womanhood." Declaring that "behind the uterus, there is a human being who suffers," he suggested that it was difficult for the physician to "help women sustain or restore their capacity to love—*to be happy and to make others happy*" (italics mine). He also demonstrated that there were few psychobiological difficulties that could compare with maternity for creating widespread suffering.[41]

In a similar vein, other medical writers cited maternity as the "fertile soil in which seeds of anxiety flourished"[42] and commented on the high incidence of mental disease in pregnant women.[43] These physicians felt the urgent need to prevent "frigid wives" and "postpartum cripples"[44] and thus to move beyond the purely "pelvic dimension" to the complex being housing the pelvis.[45] One gynecologist asserted that physicians could "reasonably assume that almost every woman will at some time develop a psychosomatic pelvic disturbance."[46] Two investigators studying thirty-three women exposed to "educated" childbirth could only find two women who classified as normal or "minimal[ly] neurotic."[47] Even such proponents of Natural Childbirth as Sawyer and Thoms readily acknowledged Deutsch as a major source of their beliefs concerning the mental and emotional life of women.[48]

Extending Deutsch's view of pregnancy as an "agent provocateur" in relation to women, some physicians viewed pregnancy as provocative in relation to themselves.[49] Indeed, psychoanalytic interpretations aimed at aiding the management of the physician-patient relationship were commonplace in midtwentieth-century professional literature concerning childbirth. Psychological writers, some of whom admitted to having little training in psychiatry or psychology, often emphasized the complex psychosexual motivations that infused the relationship between the childbearing woman and her physician.[50] A pervasive theme in the discussion of the emotional life of childbearing women was the view of women as threatening. More precisely, the childbearing woman was threatening because she invested so much libidinal energy in the pregnancy and in the physician-patient relationship.

Sawyer, citing Deutsch, described the "forces" unleashed by maternity as the "most powerful emotional processes" known to humans. The physician, in Sawyer's view, was constantly "face to face with a psychological force almost unbelievable." For Sawyer, Natural Childbirth was a "deliberate attempt to harness, direct, and control" the emotions in women that made the "world go round" but that ultimately needed controlling.[51]

Other medical wirters, using the language of psychoanalysis, were concerned with the extent to which childbearing women transferred their "libidinal fixations" to their obstetricians with their tendency to "disrobe emotionally" in their presence and with their virtually "fanatic" attachments to physicians whom they saw as father figures and gods.[52] While some physicians viewed this kind of transference as a positive factor in their relationships with obstetric patients, they were also, paradoxically, worried about the "sensual elements" in the relationship.[53]

Erik Erikson, a key figure in the development and revision of Freudian thought, criticized some physicians' tendency to interpret the childbearing woman's behavior in psychosexual terms. Specifically, Erikson objected to the undue emphasis placed on "sublimated sexual attachment to the obstetrician with a resulting interpretation of the delivery as a grandiose sex act," instead of the professional admitting that women might derive pleasure from their own mastery of childbirth and that such pleasure was healthy.[54]

If childbearing women were psychosexually threatening to some physicians, they were also suspect because they were perceived as undermining physicians' claims to expertise in obstetrics.[55] Some physician advocates of Natural Childbirth were especially concerned that those nonphysicians who proselytized the method were putting themselves between the physician and his patient, thus robbing women of their "greatest moral support."[56] Literature on prenatal advice and Natural Childbirth, in particular, written by physicians, repeatedly advised women not to engage in "bridge-table" obstetrics nor to believe what the gossiping network of women around them told them about childbirth. According to these physicians, women's eagerness to share terrible stories about childbirth was the single most important cause of women's continuing fear of childbirth. Physicians ridiculed women for viewing each other and women's magazines as legitimate sources of information about childbirth. As Natural Childbirth advocate Frederick Goodrich asserted, girls learned about reproduction from their mothers "who knew very little and consequently are poor teachers."[57]

Physicians increasingly expected nurses to provide the antepartal training and intrapartal support required in Natural Childbirth, or at least to include varying aspects of the psychosomatic approach into the care of childbearing women. But they also underscored their point that nurses could never be more than substitutes for them and, at times, poor ones. One cruel nurse could ruin everything the physician had achieved with his patient.[58] In short, women, as mothers, friends, and nurses, were often depicted as the least knowledgeable about childbirth, as sexually frustrated or embittered harridans who derived a singular pleasure from tormenting pregnant women, and as usurpers of the physician's role as chief adviser and mentor to the pregnant woman.

In the 1940s and 1950s, against the background of renewed inquiry into the emotional life of the childbearing woman

stimulated by Read and Deutsch, obstetricians and psychiatrists tended to view women as especially prone to emotional
disorders by virtue of their capacity to bear children. In their
view, even if there were no medical or obstetric complications,
childbirth could not be viewed as a truly normal state because
of the psychoneurotic tendencies that existed in virtually every
person, special varieties of which childbirth could mobilize in
women. Moreover, even if women could be considered on the
whole as psychologically as stable as men, pregnant women
could not be judged as being stable, even in relation to non-
pregnant women. While maternity did not directly cause mental illness, it was clearly a precipitating cause. Maternity re-
vived traumatic and repressed oral, anal, and genital
developmental conflicts. Pregnant women overly identified with
their fetuses, their mothers, their fathers, and even their doctors. Both pregnancy *and* the absence of pregnancy profoundly influenced women who were anxious when they were
pregnant and anxious when they were not. Most importantly,
the "happy pregnant" woman was itself a contradiction in terms
since it was virtually impossible to be completely happy while
pregnant.[59]

Although happiness in childbirth was hard to achieve,
professionals nevertheless worked toward that goal. By the end
of the 1950s, most medical training programs in obstetrics-
gynecology contained material with "a bit of psychiatric orientation."[60] Childbearing women were subject to personality
and developmental history appraisals.[61] Most importantly,
Natural Childbirth itself had acquired a distinctively psychodynamic profile. The very fact that it shared with Freudian
psychology a common interest in women's experiences of pain
and pleasure (masochism), in women's participation in childbirth (masculine activity versus female passivity), and in
women's fears in childbirth (repressed conflicts) made Natural
Childbirth subject to and thus compromised by interpretation
in psychoanalytic terms. In Read's view, pregnant women were
not abnormal nor to be suspected. In a somewhat naive psychoanalytic view, they were. Most significantly, women's quest
for pleasure in childbirth was itself suspect, as feminine masochism, narcissism, and penis envy made their way into the
Natural Childbirth dialogue.

Notes

1. Nicholson Eastman, "The Middle Road in Obstetrics," *Ladies Home Journal*, May 1952, p. 11; Charles S. Stevenson, "Obstetric Analgesia and Anesthesia: Current Problems," *Journal of the Michigan State Medical Society* 53 (August 1954):860.
2. Frederick W. Goodrich, "Experience With Natural Childbirth," *Public Health Nursing* 41 (March 1949):122–25.
3. Herbert Thoms and Emil D. Karlovsky, "Two Thousand Deliveries Under a Training for Childbirth Program: A Statistical Survey and Commentary," *American Journal of Obstetrics and Gynecology* 68 (July 1954):279–84.
4. Marion D. Laird and Margaret Hogan, "An Elective Program on Preparation for Childbirth at the Sloane Hospital for Women, May 1951 to June 1953," *American Journal of Obstetrics and Gynecology* 72 (September 1956):641–47.
5. Herbert Thoms and William C. Billings, "A Consideration of Childbirth Programs," *New England Journal of Medicine*, 1 November 1956, p. 860.
6. C. Lee Buxton, "An Evaluation of a Prepared Childbirth Program," *New York State Journal of Medicine*, 1 September 1956, p. 2660; H. Lloyd Miller, "Prenatal Training in Private Practice: Report on 2140 Consecutive Deliveries," *Obstetrics and Gynecology* 8 (October 1956):475; and H. Lloyd Miller, Francis E. Flannery, and Dorothy Bell, "Education for Childbirth in Private Practice:450 Consecutive Cases," *American Journal of Obstetrics and Gynecology* 63 (April 1952):796.
7. "Two Gynecologists Write Book for Parents-To-Be," *New York Herald Tribune*, 20 October 1950, p. 28, clipping in Thoms' scrapbooks.
8. "Doctors With Same Purpose Have Different Approaches," *West Hartford News*, 14 February 1952, clipping in Thoms' scrapbooks.
9. Thoms and Billings, "Consideration of Childbirth Programs," p. 860.
10. Lawrence Zelic Freedman and Herbert Thoms, "Observations on Training for Childbirth," *Journal of the American Medical Women's Association* 13 (January 1958):46.
11. Buxton, "Evaluation of a Prepared Childbirth Program," p. 2660; Grantly Dick-Read to Herbert Thoms,(?) 26 February 1948, private collection of Margaret Thoms.
12. "The Story of the Work of the Maternity Center Association," files of the Maternity Center Association, New York City.
13. J. H. Pollock, "The Case for Natural Childbirth," *Cosmopolitan*, July 1953, pp. 39–43.

14. Vera R. Keane, "Preparation for Labor," *Public Health Nursing* 44 (September 1952):503.

15. See note 38, chapter 4.

16. Buxton, "Evaluation of a Prepared Childbirth Program," p. 2661.

17. Paul Bowers, "Natural Childbirth," *Medical Clinics of North America* (Philadelphia: W. B. Saunders, 1955), p. 1792; C. Lee Buxton, "Prepared Childbirth and Rooming-In at Yale," *Pennsylvania Medical Journal* 60 (February 1957):172; and Sol T. DeLee and Iva J. Duncan, "Training for Natural Childbirth," *American Journal of Nursing* 56 (January 1956):48–49.

18. Interestingly enough, the drug selected was supposed to "fit" the skill of the physician. Physicians stated that the drug had to fit the patient *and* the physician, which created a conflict since not every physician was skilled in every drug regimen and, therefore, not in a position to offer every woman the best choice for her. In "Trends in Anti-Pain Drugs," *New York Times*, 13 April 1951, p. 26, a physician stated that the drug chosen should suit the patient and then stated that a physician needed to be skilled in two or three methods, implying that a woman might have a doctor who was not skilled in the method best for her.

19. Frances Kocklauner, in "Obstetrical Analgesia and Anesthesia," *Bulletin of the American Association of Nurse Anesthetists* 11 (February 1943):27–33, noted that at the University Hospitals of Cleveland, women were given morphine and scopolamine for a first labor "unless the doctor orders otherwise." The American College of Obstetricians and Gynecologists' warning in the *Manual of Standards in Obstetric-Gynecologic Practice* (Chicago: American College of Obstetricians and Gynecologists, 1959), p. 24, that "routine orders for medication are condemned," indicates that orders for medication were routine and out of the realm of choice for women.

20. Laird and Hogan, "An Elective Program," pp. 641–42; John E. Stoll, "Experiences with Natural Childbirth: Report of Two Hundred Cases from Private Practice and Public Clinic, Including Four Sets of Twins," *Western Journal of Surgery, Obstetrics and Gynecology* 59 (February 1951):50–52.

21. Buxton, "Prepared Childbirth and Rooming-In at Yale," pp. 174–76; Leon Chertok, *Motherhood and Personality: Psychosomatic Aspects of Childbirth*, trans. D. Graham (London: Tavistock, 1969) and *Psychosomatic Methods in Painless Childbirth: History, Theory and Practice*, trans. Denis Leigh (New York: Pergamon Press, 1959); and William S. Kroger, " 'Natural Childbirth': Is the Read Method of 'Natural Childbirth' Waking Hypnosis?" *Medical Times* 80 (August 1952):484–91.

22. "I Watched My Baby Born," *Pageant*, January 1949, clipping in Thoms' scrapbooks.

23. "Natural Childbirth," *Modern Romances*, August 1949, clipping in Thoms' scrapbooks.

24. Gretta Palmer, "Having Your Baby the New Way," *Collier's*, 13 November 1948, clipping in Thoms' scrapbooks; Frederick Goodrich, *Natural Childbirth: A Manual for Expectant Parents* (New York: Prentice-Hall, 1950), p. 12.

25. Dorothy Barclay, " 'Natural Childbirth': A Progress Report," *New York Times*, 29 November 1950, sec. 6, p. 34.

26. Samuel B. Kirkwood, "Twenty Years of Maternal Care," *Children* 2 (July-August 1955):136–37.

27. H. Atlee, *Natural Childbirth* (Springfield, Ill.: Charles C. Thomas, 1956); Julie Harris, as told to Betty Friedan, "I Was Afraid to Have a Baby," *McCall's*, December 1956, pp. 68–74; and Carl Tupper, "Conditioning for Childbirth," *American Journal of Obstetrics and Gynecology* 71 (April 1956):733–40.

28. Eastman, "Middle Road in Obstetrics," p. 91.

29. Barbara Gelb, *The ABC of Natural Childbirth* (New York: W. W. Norton, 1954); Margaret Gamper, *Relax: Here's Your Baby* (Chicago: Campus Service, 1951), p. 77.

30. Lucille G. Denman, "Experiences in Childbirth—A Gratifying Experience," *American Journal of Nursing* 51 (January 1951):27.

31. Robert A. Hingson and Louis M. Hellman, "Eight Thousand Parturients Evaluate Drugs, Techniques, and Doctors During Labor and Delivery: A Qualitative and Quantitative Assay of Obstetrical Amnesia, Analgesia, Anesthesia, and Psychological Lobotomy During Childbirth," *American Journal of Obstetrics and Gynecology* 68 (July 1954):262–78; Fred D. Kartchner, "A Study of the Emotional Reactions During Labor," *American Journal of Obstetrics and Gynecology* 60 (July 1950):19–29; and Norman Pleshette, Stuart S. Asch, and Janet Chase, "A Study of Anxieties During Pregnancy, Labor, the Early and Late Puerperium," *Bulletin of the New York Academy of Medicine* 32 (June 1956):436–55.

32. Grantly Dick-Read, *Introduction to Motherhood* (New York: Harper and Brothers, 1950), p. 30.

33. Ibid., p. 31.

34. Ibid., p. 4.

35. Grantly Dick-Read, *Childbirth Without Fear: The Principles and Practice of Natural Childbirth*, 2nd ed., rev. (New York: Harper and Row, Har/Row, 1970), p. 362.

36. John S. Haller and Robin M. Haller, *The Physician and Sexuality in Victorian America* (New York: W. W. Norton, 1974), pp. 80,

47–87, 131–35; George H. Napheys, *The Physical Life of Woman: Advice to the Maiden, Wife, and Mother* (Philadelphia: George MacLean, 1869).

37. Franklin S. Newell, "Anesthesia in the First Stage of Labor," *Surgery, Gynecology and Obstetrics* 3 (July 1906):126–30; Joseph B. DeLee, "The Prophylactic Forceps Operation," *Transactions of the American Gynecological Society* (Philadelphia: William J. Dornan, 1920), pp. 66–78; Roy P. Finney, *The Story of Motherhood* (New York: Liveright, 1937); and Alan Frank Guttmacher, *Into This Universe: The Story of Human Birth* (New York: Viking Press, 1937).

38. William Benbow Thompson, "Neuroses of War Wives," *California and Western Medicine* 63 (October 1945):167.

39. Helene Deutsch, *The Psychology of Women Volume II. Motherhood* (1945; reprint ed., New York: Bantam, 1973), p. 267. Grantly Dick-Read to Herbert Thoms, 1 March 1949, private collection of Margaret Thoms. Read stated that he disagreed with most of what Deutsch had to say about him and his method.

40. Ernst Simmel, "The Significance of Psychoanalysis for Gynecology," *California and Western Medicine* 63 (October 1945):169.

41. Ibid., pp. 169–71.

42. Howard C. Walser, "Fear, An Important Etiological Factor in Obstetric Problems," *American Journal of Obstetrics and Gynecology* 55 (May 1948):799–805.

43. Dwight M. Palmer, "Psychosomatic Orientations in Obstetrics and Gynecology," *Ohio State Medical Journal* 45 (October 1949):965–70.

44. Kenneth A. Podger, "Emotional Aspects of Present Day Obstetrics," *North Carolina Medical Journal* 15 (June 1954):256.

45. Freedman and Thoms, "Observations on Training for Childbirth," p. 51.

46. Arthur J. Mandy, "The Emotional Aspects of Obstetric and Gynecologic Disorders," *American Journal of Obstetrics and Gynecology* 60 (September 1950):605.

47. Patricia Donovan and Selma Landisberg, "Some Psychologic Observations of 'Educated Childbirth,'" *New York State Journal of Medicine*, 1 November 1953, p. 2504.

48. Blackwell Sawyer, "Experiences With the Labor Procedure of Grantly Dick-Read," *American Journal of Obstetrics and Gynecology* 51 (June 1946):852–58; Herbert Thoms, *Training for Childbirth: A Program of Natural Childbirth With Rooming-In* (New York: McGraw-Hill, 1950).

49. Helene Deutsch, "An Introduction to the Discussion of the Psychological Problems of Pregnancy," in *Problems of Early Infancy,*

ed. Milton J. E. Senn (New York: Josiah Macy Jr., Foundation, 1948), p. 17.

50. Willard R. Cooke, "The Differential Psychology of the American Woman," *American Journal of Obstetrics and Gynecology* 49 (April 1945):457–72.

51. Sawyer, "Experiences with the Labor Procedure," p. 852.

52. Donovan and Landisberg, "Some Psychologic Observations," p. 2505; Mandy, "Emotional Aspects," p. 606; Theodore R. Seidman, *Becoming A Mother* (New York: David McKay, 1956); and Simmel, "Significance of Psychoanalysis," p. 174.

53. Fritz Wengraf, *Psychosomatic Approach to Gynecology and Obstetrics* (Springfield, Ill.: Charles C. Thomas, 1953), pp. 190–211.

54. See the remarks following Albert M. Vollmer, "Clinical Experiences and Observations on the Use of Relaxation in Obstetrical Practice," in *Problems of Early Infancy,* ed. Milton J. E. Senn, p. 56.

55. Some clinicians, including Deutsch herself, suggested that obstetricians were themselves in conflict over their bonds with women. For example, Howard Walser, in "Some Clinical Observations on the Influence of Emotions in Pregnancy," in *Problems of Early Infancy,* p. 69, stated that obstetricians were "sublimat[ing] strong feminine components of their personalities" and were "vicariously giving birth to their own brain child" when they assisted women to give birth. Deutsch, in the *Psychology of Women,* p. 270, remarked that obstetricians were depriving women of the pleasures of maternity because of their "repressed infantile wish to give birth" themselves.

56. Harold B. Davidson, "Training for Childbirth," *Postgraduate Medicine* 25 (April 1959):457.

57. Goodrich, *Natural Childbirth,* pp. 14–15.

58. Donovan and Landisberg, "Some Psychologic Observations," p. 2505; Frederick W. Goodrich, "Modern Obstetrics and the Nurse," *American Journal of Nursing* 57 (May 1957):586–88.

59. Robert N. Crendick, "The Patient Psychologically Unprepared for Labor," *Clinical Obstetrics and Gynecology* 2 (June 1959):318.

60. Ibid., p. 320.

61. William S. Kroger, "Psychosomatic Aspects of Obstetrics and Gynecology," *Obstetrics and Gynecology* 3 (May 1954):504–16.

6 _____

EPILOGUE AND CONCLUSION: FROM PLEASURE TO CONTROL _____

By 1960, arguably little substantive change had occurred in the way most American women experienced childbirth. After his second tour of the United States in 1957, Grantly Dick-Read commented on Americans' growing interest in Natural Childbirth, but he lamented the "trend in American obstetrics toward an element of servitude to mechanization and the materialization of childbirth."[1] Struck by the paradox of a nation "so efficiently equipped for war under the pious persuasion of self-preservation and peace that war became almost inevitable," Read marveled that American hospitals had no provision for "the absence of" emergencies and complications in childbirth.[2] For Read, American maternity care in hospitals was still "kindness by incarceration."[3]

American physicians still indicated their preference for DeLee's prophylactic methods[4] and for the "whole arsenal of contemporary technology and pain relievers: the barbiturates, seconal, nembutal and amytal; the amnesic, scopolamine; the narcotic drugs, demoral [sic] and novocain; the muscle relaxant, curare; and, if necessary, the use of obstetrical forceps."[5] Medical literature continued to emphasize pharmacologic pain relief and indicated that the anesthesiologist had become almost as important to the childbearing woman as her obstetrician.[6] Nursing literature showed a greater attention to the details of providing Natural Childbirth to women but also, to a lesser extent, paralleled medical literature in the proportion of space allotted to pharmacologic pain relief.[7] In addition, nurses failed to show that they differed substantially from physicians in the value they assigned to prophylactic obstetrics or in their view of childbearing women as beset by deep psychic conflicts requiring expert intervention.

Despite Americans' continued interest in Natural Childbirth, the method, as practiced in American hospitals, had difficulty competing with pharmacologic regimens (especially those that promised painlessness and consciousness), which were really more suited to the hospital environment and the orientation of most professional attendants who still viewed childbirth as a *treatable* entity. If a psychophysical method was going to work for larger numbers of American women, it would have to offer them the means to withstand the subtle and overt pressures toward relying on drugs and instruments that existed in hospitals, and it would have to be informed by something other than a traditional view of women and the physician-patient relationship.

Psychoprophylaxis was arguably such a method. It made its way to the United States from Russia via France. Fernand Lamaze, a French obstetrician, derived his theory and method of "painless childbirth" from the experimental work of Russian scientists conducted in the 1920s and 1930s. Introduced in Russia in 1947 by a neuropsychiatrist and based on Pavlovian concepts of pain perception and conditioned reflexes, psychoprophylaxis evolved from and eventually replaced hypnosuggestive methods of pain relief in childbirth in that country.

Impressed by the systematic application of the method in Russia and by the demonstration of a painless birth in a Russian labor unit, Lamaze introduced it with several modifications in France in 1951. The method soon moved from France throughout Europe and was eventually championed in the United States by the English physiotherapist Elisabeth Bing. Most Americans probably learned of the method from Marjorie Karmel, a woman who had herself experienced two Lamaze births (one in France under Lamaze's supervision). Her book, *Thank You, Dr. Lamaze: A Mother's Experiences in Painless Childbirth*, published in 1959, introduced Lamaze since few American publications mentioned the Lamaze method before that time. After 1960, with the establishment of the American Society for Psychoprophylaxis in Obstetrics, the Lamaze method in various forms became the most popular psychophysical method of pain relief in childbirth in the United States.[8]

Although much more heavily couched in the language of neurophysiology than Read's presentation of Natural Childbirth, the Lamaze method was indistinguishable from Natural Childbirth in virtually every major respect (theory, method, and goals). While Read, Lamaze, and their respective followers certainly argued about the originality and uniqueness of these methods, both of them included similar didactic, psychotherapeutic, and physiotherapeutic elements.[9] What appeared distinctive about the Lamaze method was its greater emphasis on women's activity and control in childbirth. For example, Lamaze asserted that women should never "cease to be the force which directs, controls, and regulates . . . labor." He also charged Read with having relegated women to "second place" in childbirth, instead of securing them in the first place where they belonged. For Lamaze, the Read method was too dependent on the physician's ability to create a state of "mystic exaltation" in his patient. Acting on his belief that civilization had ruined the experience of childbirth for women, Read, in Lamaze's opinion, asked his patient to "decivilize" herself by yielding to the ecstasy of childbirth. While ecstasy, provided it was achieved, might act as a positive influence in labor, the "relaxation," "dulling of consciousness," and passivity that the Read method also required acted as negative influences.[10] For Lamaze, control, not pleasure per se, was the central guiding principle in childbirth.

In effect, Lamaze suggested that the Read method was more metaphysical than scientific, and he conveyed his belief that Natural Childbirth attempted to turn a woman on to her labor at the same time that it attempted to tune her out of awareness of it. By dissociating herself from her body, instead of focusing on its sensations, the laboring woman ended up submitting to them, not acting with them. According to Lamaze, Read's patient was *entranced* with her physician and the idea of giving birth, while Lamaze's patient *acted* to give birth. Lamaze implied that Read's patient was no better off and no more in control of the childbirth process or herself than the woman who received a regional block anesthetic, which also dissociated a woman from the sensations of childbirth and placed her under the influence of the physician.

Marjorie Karmel also established the difference between the Read and Lamaze methods of childbirth by emphasizing women's activity and control (self-control and control of the conduct of childbirth). In her view, the Read patient passively allowed nature to take its course in labor while the Lamaze patient was trained to defy nature with her own mental and physical resources. The Lamaze method was not "natural" childbirth at all, but rather it was "better" than nature. The Lamaze patient was trained like an athlete to make her body obey her *against* the commands nature sent her, such as the urge to push. In contrast to the Read patient, The Lamaze patient's mind was never at rest, even if her body was. (In the Twilight Sleep argument, the patient's mind was perceived as resting while the body actively contended with nature.)

Appearing throughout her book as a strong and forceful woman, Karmel suggested why the Lamaze method might have held more appeal than the Read method to the woman who derived pleasure from control and less appeal to the physician who saw himself as properly in control of events in the labor room. Significantly, she noted the difficulty women had in freely participating in childbirth while subjected to hospital routines and the importance American physicians seemed to place on the "psychological" relationship between the doctor and his patient, which some physicians saw as being endangered by the Lamaze method. Most importantly, Karmel stated that the "proof" for the method lay not in its "theoretical logic" but rather in its effectiveness in actual practice. Karmel implied that the well-trained Lamaze patient had a better chance to achieve her goals in childbirth than the Read patient, no matter what the circumstances were.[11]

Physicians demonstrated that they were not unaware of the challenge of a method that promised safety, pleasure, and control (in terms of self-mastery and control of the management of childbirth) without the use of drugs and instruments and, therefore, conceivably *without physicians*. Indeed, the idea that a woman might be so "thrilled" to play an "active" role in childbirth that she forgot that the doctor was "of utmost importance" had been expressed in relation to the Read method.[12] Americans' interest in yet another childbirth method that did not inherently require physicians for its use and their continuing dissatisfaction with hospital maternity care provoked continuing "dis-ease" among physicians. Moreover, they persisted in coping with this "dis-ease" by depicting women as threatening and any childbirth regimen not in physician control as unsafe.

For example, two physicians saw women's dissatisfaction with prevailing obstetric practices as a problem of "public relations." Women now took safety in childbirth for granted and failed to give "special credit to the medical profession which is responsible" for it. Furthermore, it was, for these physicians, an "enigma of modern obstetrics that what passes in the record as a normal labor and delivery may be bitterly remembered by our patients as a terrifying experience."[13] More significantly, nurses were the ones who most influenced the satisfaction of maternity patients. Specifically, if nurses did not properly execute their function of public relations for physicians and hospitals, the result was unhappy patients. "No nurse should ever be described as sarcastic, hostile, scolding, or impatient." Patients did not pay high fees for hospital care only to be "berated" by nurses. In the opinion of these physicians, women's own tendency to evaluate obstetric care by criteria other than safety and nurses' treatment of women in hospitals were the key factors in the rise of alternative childbirth regimens.[14]

Louis Hellman, a prominent obstetrician, acknowledged in 1962 that patients were not satisfied with their doctors but asserted that no one could deny "the commonsense fact that the mothers of America would be better off if each at the time of labor and delivery were continuously attended by a Board-certified obstetrician."[15] Concerned about the public's "increased search for a panacea hopefully to be found in the 'isms' of natural or psychoprophylactic childbirth," Hellman, nevertheless, assured his colleagues that these were nothing more than "small clouds" on the "beautiful horizon" of decreasing maternal and infant deaths and the "satisfying and lucrative practice" of obstetrics.[16] He also expressed his ambivalence about nurses by acknowledging the need for them to "extend the hand" of the obstetrician but also by admitting how "unpalatable" this was. Hellman was clearly concerned that the nurse "double" the activities of the physician, without "downgrad[ing]" or "supplant[ing]" him and without escaping "continuing physician control."[17]

A more comprehensive illustration of some physicians' discomfort with Americans' interest in drug-free methods of childbirth is Waldo Fielding's *The Childbirth Challenge: Commonsense Versus "Natural" Methods*. In the book, published in 1962, Fielding, with the help of one of his former patients, attempted to show that all "natural" methods were dangerous to American democracy and the American woman's mind. His critique shows the importance of the feminine mystique and the Cold War in rationalizing some physicians' fears about childbirth methods that could be employed without them. Emphasizing the Soviet origins of the Lamaze method, which he tied to the Read method, and questioning the motivations and general emotional stability of American women who were attracted to these methods, Fielding dismissed them as dangerous "propaganda."[18]

Other literature also continued to emphasize that any woman who elected to experience a "natural" method was herself suspect and that it was not only nonsensical for women to use these methods but also unsafe and unwise for everyone concerned—themselves, their husbands, their babies, their physicians, and American society as a whole.[19] These critics did not doubt that childbirth, "even in 1961, is a cataclysmic upheaval of nature" requiring unnatural solutions.[20]

The Legacy of Natural Childbirth

The Natural Childbirth dialogue showed elements of both change and continuity in Americans' attitudes toward and conduct of childbirth. First, Natural Childbirth, like other pain-relieving regimens, showed professionals' continuing preoccupation with the pain of labor and delivery and not with the commonly occurring pains, for example, from episiotomy, breast engorgement, or uterine "afterpains." While women often suffer these pains even more intensely than the pain of labor, the prevention and treatment of pain in obstetrics continued to focus on the labor and delivery period. Women clearly expressed their greatest anxieties about this period, but it is also clear that labor and delivery was what physicians prized the most about maternity and the responsibility for which they were most reluctant to delegate to anyone else. The climactic, life-and-death nature of childbirth seemed to best legitimate the physician's role in obstetrics. Prior to the invention and widespread use of diagnostic and therapeutic technologies aimed at the fetus in the prenatal period, labor and delivery was the event most subject to medical intervention.

Second, Natural Childbirth, like the Twilight Sleep, separated pain from the fear of pain and the sensation of pain from the evaluative context in which it was experienced.[21] In both the Twilight Sleep and Natural Childbirth, the fear of childbirth pain was the target of treatment or prevention. In the Twilight Sleep, pain was "good" when it occurred but "bad" if a woman was aware of it. In Natural Childbirth, pain was not "so bad" or "hurt so good" if a woman was not afraid of it and did not necessarily exist at all if a woman did not anticipate it. Moreover, both methods prescribed a specific physical and psychological context for birth-giving. A successful birth by Twilight Sleep or Natural Childbirth required skilled and supportive caregivers with a positive attitude toward the methods and a controlled, subdued environment. Yet, unlike Twilight Sleep and other drug regimens, Natural Childbirth promised a relatively drug-free solution to the problem of pain and did not start with the presumption that childbirth was painful at all.

Third, Natural Childbirth shifted the emphasis in obstetrics from an exclusive concern for women's safety to their satisfaction or pleasure in childbirth and, therefore, altered the criteria against which obstetric outcomes were measured. In fact, Natural Childbirth legitimated the consideration of "soft" outcomes, such as self-fulfillment and happiness, in all cases of childbirth, "natural" or controlled with drugs. When medical safety was the sole concern, criteria relating to the physiological course of labor and morbidity and mortality rates determined if an outcome was evaluated positively or negatively. An outcome was "good" if mother and child survived childbirth without physical injury. Natural Childbirth forced a new "calculus"—a new mandate to balance safety requirements with women's desire to be happy in childbirth. An outcome was now "successful" if mother and child emerged from childbirth safely *and* if the childbearing woman was happy with herself and her childbirth experience, if she was able to control her behavior in labor and cooperate with her caregivers, with or without the aid of drugs, and if she returned to the same obstetrician for a second pregnancy.[22]

While professionals used to be concerned with the safety of using drugs and instruments versus the safety of not using them—safety being the sole criterion—after 1948, professionals had to balance safety with satisfaction. When was it proper to subordinate a factor of safety to one of satisfaction, if ever? What happened when the professional, who always gave more weight to safety, encountered a patient who weighed safety and satisfaction equally or gave greater weight to the latter? The current debate concerning home birth illustrates well the continuing conflict between the needs for safety and satisfaction in childbirth, which separate professionals from childbearing women.

Fourth, with the advent of Natural Childbirth, pain was no longer exclusively located in the action of uterine muscles, the dilatation of the cervix, and the stretching of the perineum but rather in the hearts and minds of women. Accordingly, the prevention or treatment of pain had to start with women themselves—the person behind the uterus. Childbirth pain became a more inclusive phenomenon, encompassing virtually all aspects of the childbearing woman's biography. While the new attention to the psychosomatic elements of childbirth humanized the birth process and engendered a new intimacy between the childbearing woman and her caregiver, it also placed her under more intensive and ultimately more intrusive professional scrutiny than ever before. What did the professional now not have a right and a duty to appraise in the interests of maternal well-being?[23]

Fifth, while increasing professional attention in the 1940s and 1950s was given to the effects of various pain-relieving regimens in childbirth on the fetus and newborn infant, the focus of Natural Childbirth remained on women and, more particularly, on their safety and happiness in childbirth.[24] Investigative reports on Natural Childbirth employed criteria almost exclusively in relation to women and the labor itself.[25] Natural Childbirth was not a response to the "discovery" of the fetus as a treatable patient since the fetus could not have been discovered in that sense until after 1960 when diagnostic and therapeutic technologies exclusively directed toward fetal welfare were in widespread use. Moreover, it was not until the 1970s that professionals paid such painstaking and "scientific" attention to the infant's postdelivery biological and behavioral responses and its ability to "bond" with its mother as functions of the amounts and kinds of anesthesia and analgesia used in labor and delivery. Natural Childbirth, with its emphasis on making women happy with themselves and their caregivers, and the rise of the fetus to independent patient status, a direct result of the invention and widespread use of fetal technologies, may be viewed as physicians' attempts to maintain control of the childbirth arena (by keeping women happy with their doctors and by finding a new patient to treat now that maternal mortality rates are so low). The motive force behind the early Natural Childbirth movement was not concern for the fetus or newborn infant per se, except as each benefited from the new attention to its mother's welfare and happiness.[26]

Sixth, Natural Childbirth showed that women could be trained to be happy even when the substantive elements of childbirth had changed very little. A woman could still be pleased under the influence of drugs and with the assistance of instruments provided she was properly "educated" or "prepared." In fact, Natural Childbirth, by not clearly differentiating itself from childbirth controlled with drugs, paradoxically demonstrated that it was not any specific regimen that ensured a happy and safe mother but rather her caregiver's attitude toward her and willingness to treat her like a person, not a repository of reproductive organs.

Finally, Natural Childbirth, in the 1940s and 1950s, was distinctively nonfeminist, if not antifeminist, and promedical in control of the childbirth arena. It is simply inaccurate to politicize the early Natural Childbirth movement by depicting women and physicians as adversaries on two sides of the Natural Childbirth argument. The trend toward psychosomatic medicine and women's increasing demand to be satisfied in childbirth converged in the Natural Childbirth movement. In the 1940s and 1950s, there were no claims made to reproductive or other "rights" in relation to childbirth, unless it was the right to be happy; and there was no clash between professionals and women over expertise in obstetrics or control of childbirth per se. Childbearing women simply wanted to be satisfied in childbirth and to be treated more humanely by their caregivers, and it was certainly in physicians' interest to help them achieve this. Moreover, it was in line with the pronatalist sentiments of the times to keep women happy to have babies.

Neither childbearing women nor nurses ever claimed greater expertise than physicians in childbirth by virtue of being women, nor did they see themselves as having the final authority in childbirth-related matters. In the age of the feminine mystique, it was right and natural that physicians assume the leadership role in childbirth.

Although the Natural Childbirth movement had the potential for being a revolutionary one, it lacked the social and political activism of the 1960s and 1970s, which emphasized women's rights, consumerism, and the demystification of the professions, as opposed to the feminine mystique and the mystique of professionalism. Moreover, by arguing against Natural Childbirth as well as assimilating it into prevailing obstetric practice, physicians succeeded in "medicalizing" and neutralizing the Natural Childbirth momentum. Accordingly, the 1960s arguably marked the dividing line between two different, but certainly related, movements—one emphasizing the pleasure of childbirth and the other emphasizing women's ultimate control of childbirth. The resolution of the second movement is yet to be determined.

Notes

1. Grantly Dick-Read, *Childbirth Without Fear*, 4th ed., rev., ed. Helen Wessel and Harlan F. Ellis (New York: Harper and Row, Perennial Library, 1979), p. 342.

2. Ibid., pp. 341–42.

3. Ibid., p. 344.

4. Clyde L. Randall, "Childbirth Without Fear of Interference," *Clinical Obstetrics and Gynecology* 2 (June 1959):360–66.

5. Natalie Gittelson, "The Case Against Natural Childbirth," *Harper's Bazaar*, February 1961, p. 137.

6. See the foreword by Robert Hingson to "Obstetric Anesthesia and Analgesia," *Clinical Obstetrics and Gynecology* 4 (March 1961):11–14.

7. See Ernestine Wiedenbach, *Family-Centered Maternity Nursing* (New York: G. P. Putnam's Sons, 1958), in contrast to other nursing texts, which allotted more space to drug regimens.

8. Leon Chertok, *Motherhood and Personality: Psychosomatic Aspects of Childbirth*, trans. D. Graham (London: Tavistock, 1969); Marjorie Karmel, *Thank You, Dr. Lamaze: A Mother's Experiences in Painless Childbirth* (Philadelphia: J. B. Lippincott, 1959); and Fernand Lamaze, *Painless Childbirth: The Lamaze Method*, trans. L. R. Celestin (New York: Henry Regnery, Pocket Books, 1972).

9. Chertok, *Motherhood and Personality*, pp. 1–21; Colleen Conway, "Psychophysical Preparations for Childbirth," in *Contemporary Obstetric and Gynecologic Nursing*, ed. L. McNall (St. Louis: C. V. Mosby, 1980), pp. 40–56; Lamaze, *Painless Childbirth*, pp. 29–30, 72–75; and Read, *Childbirth Without Fear*, 4th ed., pp. 324–32.

10. Lamaze, *Painless Childbirth*, pp. 29–30, 72–75.

11. Karmel, *Thank You, Dr. Lamaze*.

12. M. Anderson, "A Fresh Look at Natural Childbirth," *Parents Magazine*, November 1956, p. 92.

13. Purvis L. Martin and Steward H. Smith, "Public Relations in Our Maternity Wards," *American Journal of Obstetrics and Gynecology* 81 (June 1961):1079.

14. Ibid., pp. 1079–85. This includes a discussion by other physicians.

15. Louis M. Hellman, "Paraobstetric Personnel," *American Journal of Obstetrics and Gynecology*, 15 February 1962, p. 503.

16. Ibid.

17. Ibid., pp. 503–7.

18. Waldo Fielding and L. Benjamin, *The Childbirth Challenge: Commonsense Versus "Natural" Methods* (New York: Viking Press, 1962).

19. Gittelson, "Case Against Natural Childbirth," pp. 136–37, 178–80; L. Robinson, "How to Know When You're Really Feminine," *Good Housekeeping*, June 1960, pp. 92–93, 162–63.

20. Gittelson, "Case Against Natural Childbirth," p. 178.

21. On the two meanings of pain, see H. T. Engelhardt, "Ethical Issues in Pain Management," in *Pain and Society*, ed. H. W. Kosterlitz and L. Y. Terenius (Weinheim: Verlag Chemie GmbH., 1980), pp. 461–67; C. S. Lewis, *The Problem of Pain* (New York: Macmillan, 1962), p. 90.

22. Natural Childbirth proponents added the terms "success" and "failure" to the dialogue about childbirth, even though they also clearly objected to their use in relation to childbearing women.

23. William Ray Arney and Jane Neill, "The Location of Pain in Childbirth: Natural Childbirth and the Transformation of Obstetrics," *Sociology of Health and Illness* 4 (1982):1–24.

24. Louis M. Hellman and Robert A. Hingson, "The Effect of Various Methods of Obstetric Pain Relief on Infant Mortality," *New York State Journal of Medicine*, 1 December 1953, pp. 2767–71.

25. See the section "Natural Childbirth versus Childbirth with Drugs" in chapter 4.

26. For a divergent view, see William Ray Arney, *Power and the Profession of Obstetrics* (Chicago: University of Chicago Press, 1982), pp. 208–42.

BIBLIOGRAPHICAL ESSAY ___

The major participants in the American dialogue concerning child-birth between 1914 and 1960 were childbearing women, physicians, and nurses. This study is, accordingly, based on evidence that shows their beliefs and practices concerning childbirth *during* that time period. Oral accounts (particularly of Natural Childbirth experiences), in which individuals look back from a vantage point in the present, were deliberately excluded for the purposes of this study since its intention was to capture the past, uninfluenced by the current debate about childbirth. More precisely, it is clear, even in published literature, that there is an unwarranted tendency to view the movement to "naturalize" childbirth, from its American beginnings in the 1940s to the present, as one movement informed by *current* beliefs and goals.

Physicians emerge as the most articulate group of the three major participants since their views appear not only in medical literature but also in nursing and popular literature. In contrast, while nurses occasionally published material in medical and popular literature, their views are primarily found in nursing literature. The group that emerges as the least articulate is childbearing women who left few firsthand accounts of their views and experiences. Attempts were made to obtain materials such as unpublished "letters to the editor" of popular magazines, women's responses on evaluation questionnaires given them during their hospital stay, and other personal documents, but these were not available. Many of these items were discarded long ago, and women were simply less likely to record their personal experiences in childbirth than professionals were to record their clinical experiences and professional beliefs.

What follows is a brief review of the types of materials used in this study, which have already been detailed in the body of the text. It is intended to provide the reader with some direction by organizing materials into useful, but certainly not inclusive, categories.

Professional Books and Journals

Professional literature, written primarily by nurses and physicians, is the richest source of data for a study such as this one. Moreover, it includes both *prescriptions* for changes in values and practices and *descriptions* of prevailing ones. Both national and regional medical, nursing, and health-related journals were located through the *Index Medicus, Cumulative Index of Nursing Literature, Nursing Studies Index*, and other indexes of this kind.

Literature was specifically sought on the topics of obstetric anesthesia and analgesia, psychophysical methods of pain relief in childbirth, including hypnosis, psychosomatic medicine, the medical and nursing care of childbearing women, and trends in obstetric care, including demographic data and statistical information on morbidity and mortality. Treatises, investigative reports, and anecdotal accounts of clinical experiences were considered.

Continuity and change in maternity care can be captured in journals as well as in successive editions of major medical and nursing texts. These included, but were not limited to, Joseph B. DeLee, *Obstetrics for Nurses*, 5th and 10th eds., rev. (Philadelphia: W. B. Saunders, 1918 and 1933); M. Edward Davis and Mabel C. Carmon, *DeLee's Obstetrics for Nurses*, 14th ed. (Philadelphia: W. B. Saunders, 1947); Joseph B. DeLee, *The Principles and Practice of Obstetrics*, 2nd–7th eds. (Philadelphia: W. B. Saunders, 1915, 1920, 1925, 1929, 1933, and 1938); Joseph B. DeLee and J. P. Greenhill, *The Principles and Practice of Obstetrics*, 8th–10th eds. and 12th ed. (Philadelphia: W. B. Saunders, 1943, 1947, 1951, and 1960); Carolyn Conant Van Blarcom, *Obstetrical Nursing*, 1st–3rd eds. and 4th ed., rev. by Erna Ziegel (New York: Macmillan, 1922, 1928, 1936, and 1957); J. Whitridge Williams, *Obstetrics: A Textbook for the Use of Students and Practitioners*, 4th–6th eds. (New York: D. Appleton, 1917, 1925, and 1930); Nicholson Eastman and Louis M. Hellman, *Williams Obstetrics*, 11th and 12th eds. (New York: Appleton-Century-Crofts, 1956 and 1961); Louise Zabriskie, *Nurses Handbook of Obstetrics*, 1st, 4th, 5th, and 6th eds. (Philadelphia: J. B. Lippincott, 1929, 1934, 1937, and 1940); and Louise Zabriskie and Nicholson Eastman, *Nurses Handbook of Obstetrics*, 9th ed. (Philadelphia: J. B. Lippincott, 1952).

Useful medical texts on pharmacologic pain relief include John J. Bonica, *The Management of Pain* (Philadelphia: Lea and Febiger, 1953); Carl Henry Davis, *Painless Childbirth Eutocia and Nitrous Oxid-Oxygen Analgesia* (Chicago: Forbes, 1916); Alfred M. Hellman, *Amnesia and Analgesia in Parturition* (New York: Paul B. Hoeber, 1915); Bert B. Hershenson, *Obstetrical Anesthesia: Its Principles and Practice* (Springfield: Ill.: Charles C. Thomas, 1955); Clifford B. Lull and Robert A. Hingson, *Control of Pain in Childbirth: Anesthesia, Analgesia, Amnesia* (Philadelphia: J. B. Lippincott, 1944); and Franklin F. Snyder, *Obstetric Analgesia and Anesthesia: Their Effects Upon Labor and the Child* (Philadelphia: W. B. Saunders, 1949).

Also useful is literature on professional curricula, such as Committee on Education of the National League for Nursing Education, *Standard Curriculum for Schools of Nursing*, 1st, 4th, and 7th eds., rev. (New York: National League for Nursing Education, 1919, 1922, and 1927); Committee on Curriculum of the National League for Nursing Education, *A Curriculum Guide for Schools of Nursing*, 2nd ed., rev. (New York: National League for Nursing Education, 1937); John Foote, comp. and ed., *State Board Questions and Answers for Nurses: Being the Actual Questions Submitted at the Examinations of 31 State Examining Boards for Nurses, With Answers*, 1st and 7th eds. (Philadelphia: J. B. Lippincott, 1917 and 1929); *State Board Questions and Answers for Nurses: Essay and Objective Types*, 17th, 19th, 20th, and 22nd eds. (Philadelphia: J. B. Lippincott, 1939, 1941, 1942, and 1944).

Popular Books, Magazines, and Newspapers

This literature includes prenatal advice books, accounts of specific childbirth regimens such as the Twilight Sleep and Natural Childbirth, and general information on pregnancy and childbirth written for the public as well as personal accounts by women of their childbirth experiences. General interest literature, such as *Time, Newsweek*, and the *New York Times*, and literature specifically directed at women, such as *Good Housekeeping, Ladies Home Journal*, and *Parents Magazine*, were considered. Indexes to newspapers, such as *New York Times Index*, and to the popular literature were most helpful. In addition, the Maternity Center Association of New York in New York City has a good collection of prenatal advice literature spanning the period of this study, but many of these books can be found in local public libraries.

Biographies and Personal Accounts

Useful were Abigail Lewis, *An Interesting Condition: The Diary of a Pregnant Woman* (Garden City, N.Y.: Doubleday, 1950); D. N. Danforth, "Contemporary Titans: Joseph Bolivar DeLee and John Whitridge Williams," *American Journal of Obstetrics and Gynecology*, 1 November 1974, pp. 577–88; Morris Fishbein with Sol Theron DeLee, *Joseph Bolivar DeLee: Crusading Obstetrician* (New York: E. P. Dutton, 1949); Frederick C. Irving, *Safe Deliverance* (Boston: Houghton Mifflin, 1942); and H. Noyes Thomas, *Doctor Courageous: The Story of Dr. Grantly Dick-Read* (Melbourne: William Heinemann, 1957).

Histories of Obstetrics and Anesthesia

These should be read as both factual accounts or secondary sources of past events and as primary sources of physicians' beliefs and values. These histories, written primarily by physicians, glorify the role of the physician and view medical innovations as progressive and "good." Palmer Findley, *Priests of Lucina: The Story of Obstetrics* (Boston: Little, Brown, 1939); Palmer Findley, *The Story of Childbirth* (Garden City, N.Y.: Doubleday, Doran, 1933); Roy P. Finney, *The Story of Motherhood* (New York: Liveright, 1937); Harvey Graham, *Eternal Eve: The History of Gynaecology and Obstetrics* (Garden City, N.Y.: Doubleday, 1951); Alan Frank Guttmacher, *Into This Universe: The Story of Human Birth* (New York: Viking Press, 1937); Howard W. Haggard, *Devils, Drugs, and Doctors: The Story of the Science of Healing From Medicine-Man to Doctor* (New York: Harper and Brothers, 1929); and Victor Robinson, *Victory Over Pain: A History of Anesthesia* (New York: Henry Schuman, 1946).

Recent Scholarship on Childbirth in America

This literature serves as a counterpoint to older histories of obstetrics and is primarily interdisciplinary in nature. Included for consideration were Joyce Antler and Daniel Fox, "The Movement Toward A Safe Maternity: Physician Accountability in New York City, 1915–1940," in *Sickness and Health in America: Readings in the History of Medicine and Public Health*, ed., Judith Walzer and Ronald Numbers (Madison: University of Wisconsin Press, 1978), pp. 375–92; Neal Devitt, "The Statistical Case for Elimination of the Midwife: Fact Versus Prejudice, 1890–1935 Part 1 and 2," *Women and Health* 4 (Spring and Summer 1979):81–96 and 169–86; Neal Devitt, "The Transition From Home to Hospital Birth in the United States, 1930–

1960," *Birth and the Family Journal* 4 (Summer 1977):47–58; Jane Donegan, "Man-Midwifery and the Delicacy of the Sexes," in *"Remember the Ladies": New Perspectives on Women in American History*, ed. Carol George (Syracuse: Syracuse University Press, 1975), pp. 90–109; Nancy Schrom Dye, "History of Childbirth in America," *Signs: Journal of Women in Culture and Society* 6 (Autumn 1980):97–108; Judith Walzer Leavitt, "Birthing and Anesthesia: The Debate Over Twilight Sleep," *Signs: Journal of Women in Culture and Society* 6 (Autumn 1980):147–64; Lawrence G. Miller, "Pain, Parturition, and the Profession: Twilight Sleep in America," in *Health Care in America: Essays in Social History*, ed. Susan Reverby and David Rosner (Philadelphia: Temple University Press, 1979), pp. 19–44; Catherine M. Scholten, " 'On the Importance of the Obstetrick Art': Changing Customs of Childbirth in America, 1760–1825," *William and Mary Quarterly* 34 (July 1977):426–45; William Ray Arney, *Power and the Profession of Obstetrics* (Chicago: University of Chicago Press, 1982); Jane B. Donegan, *Women and Men Midwives: Medicine, Morality, and Misogyny in Early America* (Westport, Conn.: Greenwood Press, 1978); Judy Barrett Litoff, *American Midwives: 1860 to the Present* (Westport, Conn.: Greenwood Press, 1978); and Richard W. Wertz and Dorothy C. Wertz, *Lying-In: A History of Childbirth in America* (New York: Free Press, 1977).

Recent Scholarship on Women

There is a large and still emerging body of literature on women informed by the new focus on women as central, rather than marginal, subjects of inquiry. Useful for this study were Jill Conway, "Women Reformers and American Culture, 1870–1930," *Journal of Social History* 5 (Winter 1971–72):164–77; Lois W. Banner, *Women in Modern America: A Brief History* (New York: Harcourt Brace Jovanovich, 1974); G. J. Barker-Benfield, *The Horrors of the Half-Known Life: Male Attitudes Toward Women and Sexuality in Nineteenth-Century America* (New York: Harper Colophon Books, 1977); William H. Chafe, *The American Woman: Her Changing Social, Economic, and Political Roles, 1920–1970* (London: Oxford University Press, 1972); Barbara Ehrenreich and Deirdre English, *For Her Own Good: 150 Years of the Experts' Advice to Women* (Garden City, N.Y.: Anchor Press/Doubleday, 1978); Sheila M. Rothman, *Woman's Proper Place: A History of Changing Ideals and Practices, 1870 to the Present* (New York: Basic Books, 1978); and June Sochen, *Movers and Shakers: American Women Thinkers and Activists, 1900–1970* (New York: Quadrangle/New York Times Book, 1973).

On the Professions of Medicine and Nursing

There is a vast literature on these professions written by their members and by outside observers, most notably in the fields of sociology and history. Most helpful here were Jo Ann Ashley, *Hospitals, Paternalism, and the Role of the Nurse* (New York: Teachers College Press, 1976); E. Richard Brown, *Rockefeller Medicine Men: Medicine and Capitalism in America* (Berkeley: University of California Press, 1979); James G. Burrow, *Organized Medicine in the Progressive Era: The Move Toward Monopoly* (Baltimore: Johns Hopkins University Press, 1977); Fred Davis, ed., *The Nursing Profession: Five Sociological Essays* (New York: John Wiley and Sons, 1966); John S. Haller and Robin M. Haller, *The Physician and Sexuality in Victorian America* (New York: W. W. Norton, 1977); Barbara Melosh, *"The Physician's Hand": Work Culture and Conflict in American Nursing* (Philadelphia: Temple University Press, 1982); Stanley Joel Reiser, *Medicine and the Reign of Technology* (Cambridge: Cambridge University Press, 1978); and Rosemary Stevens, *American Medicine and the Public Interest* (New Haven: Yale University Press, 1971).

On the Concepts of Pain and Pleasure

Most helpful in understanding pain and pleasure were David Bakan, *Disease, Pain, and Suffering: Toward A Psychology of Suffering* (Chicago: University of Chicago Press, 1968); Daniel De Moulin, "A Historical-Phenomenological Study of Bodily Pain in Western Man," *Bulletin of the History of Medicine* 48 (Winter 1974):540–70; Shizuko Y. Fagerhaugh and Anselm Strauss, *Politics of Pain Management: Staff-Patient Interaction* (Menlo Park, Calif.: Addison-Wesley, 1977); H. W. Kosterlitz and L. Y. Terenius, eds., *Pain and Society* (Weinheim: Verlag Chemie GmbH., 1980); C. S. Lewis, *The Problem of Pain* (New York: Macmillan, 1962); K. L. Norr et al., "Explaining Pain and Enjoyment in Childbirth," *Journal of Health and Social Behavior* 18 (September 1977):260–75; Martin Steven Pernick, "A Calculus of Suffering: Pain, Anesthesia, and Utilitarian Professionalism in Nineteenth Century American Medicine" (Ph.D. dissertation, Columbia University, 1979); Richard Serjeant, *The Spectrum of Pain* (London: Rupert Hart-Davis, 1969); Richard A. Sternbach, *Pain: A Psychophysiological Analysis* (New York: Academic Press, 1968); Thomas S. Szasz, *Pain and Pleasure: A Study of Bodily Feelings* (New York: Basic Books, 1957); and Mark Zborowski, *People in Pain* (San Francisco: Jossey-Bass, 1969).

Unpublished Materials

Most useful were the four scrapbooks of newspaper and magazine clippings and personal mementos left by Herbert Thoms and now located at the Yale Medical History Library in New Haven. Also important was the private collection of letters generously shared by Margaret Thoms, Herbert Thoms' daughter. These include correspondence with Grantly Dick-Read and others concerning Thoms' involvement with Natural Childbirth. The Maternity Center Association of New York houses an excellent library on childbirth materials which includes pamphlets and uncatalogued notes for lectures and addresses. The association minutes and other organizational materials are not yet available to the public.

Other useful collections—such as the minutes of the Ohio Obstetrical Society and an unpublished address by Calvina MacDonald, a nursing director of the women's division of University Hospitals of Cleveland (now called MacDonald House)—are located in the Cleveland Health Sciences Library, Historical Division and the Hospital Archives, respectively.

INDEX ————————————————

About the Author

MARGARETE SANDELOWSKI is Assistant Professor and Coordinator of the Graduate Program in Parent-Child Health Nursing at the Louisiana State University Medical Center School of Nursing. Her previous writings include *Women, Health, and Choice* and articles in *American Journal of Maternal-Child Nursing* and *Journal of Obstetric, Gynecologic, and Neonatal Nursing*.